# Bridging Biology and Behavior in Autism - Innovations in Research and Practice

*Edited by Marco Carotenuto and Carola Costanza*

Published in London, United Kingdom

Bridging Biology and Behavior in Autism - Innovations in Research and Practice
http://dx.doi.org/10.5772/intechopen.1006440
Edited by Marco Carotenuto and Carola Costanza

Contributors
Davide Marocco, Deepa Azhchath Vasu, Gerit Pfuhl, Jihad Torky, Joby Pulikkan, Leif Ekblad, Mottakunja Deepthi, Nagehan Bilgeç, Nitza Weinstein, Noury Bakrim, Roberta Simeoli, Tony Grace, Waganesh A. Zeleke



First published in London, United Kingdom, 2025 by IntechOpen
IntechOpen is the global imprint of INTECHOPEN LIMITED, registered in England and Wales, registration number: 11086078, 167-169 Great Portland Street, London, W1W 5PF, United Kingdom

For EU product safety concerns: IN TECH d.o.o., Prolaz Marije Krucifikse Kozulić 3, 51000 Rijeka, Croatia, info@intechopen.com or visit our website at intechopen.com.

British Library Cataloguing-in-Publication Data
A catalogue record for this book is available from the British Library

Bridging Biology and Behavior in Autism - Innovations in Research and Practice
Edited by Marco Carotenuto and Carola Costanza
p. cm.
Print ISBN 978-1-83634-839-9
Online ISBN 978-1-83634-838-2
eBook (PDF) ISBN 978-1-83634-840-5

If disposing of this product, please recycle the paper responsibly.

# Meet the editor

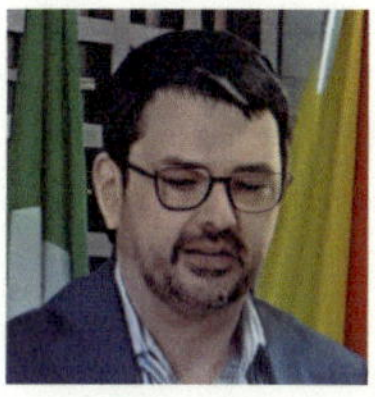

Marco Carotenuto, M. D., Ph.D., M. S., is a Full Professor of Child Neuropsychiatry at the University of Campania "Luigi Vanvitelli" in Italy, where he also directs the Child Neuropsychiatry Unit. He earned his medical degree there in 2000, specialized in Child Neuropsychiatry in 2005 after completing clinical training in the UK, and obtained a Ph.D. in Behavioral Sciences and Learning Disorders in 2008. Appointed Full Professor in 2018, he leads in both academia and clinical practice. Since 2022, he has served as President of the National Commission for Neurotherapy and Psychomotor Therapy in Developmental Age (TNPEE) and directs the School of Specialization in Child Neuropsychiatry. Author of over 300 publications, his work focuses on autism, sleep disturbances, headaches, epilepsy, and neurocognitive rehabilitation in children.

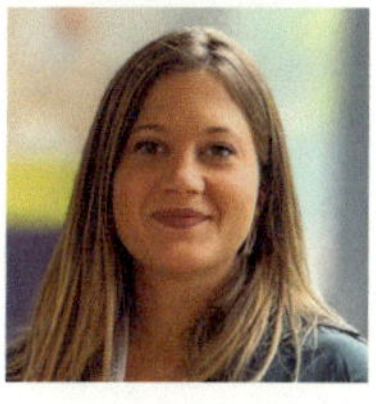

Carola Costanza, M. D., is a Child and Adolescent Neuropsychiatrist and Ph.D. Student in Health Promotion and Cognitive Sciences at the University of Palermo, Italy. After earning her medical degree from Sapienza University of Rome, she began her specialization in Child Neuropsychiatry with a strong clinical and research focus on neurodevelopmental disorders, digital addictions, and neuroinflammation. She currently works at the IRCCS Oasi Research Institute in Troina, where she is involved in the diagnosis and treatment of autism spectrum disorder, ADHD, intellectual disability, communication and motor disorders, genetic syndromes, and epilepsy. Dr. Costanza also serves as a reviewer for peer-reviewed journals in the field of child neuropsychiatry and neuroscience, and actively contributes to multidisciplinary clinical and academic research.

# Contents

# Preface

*Bridging Biology and Behavior in Autism – Innovations in Research and Practice* is a multidisciplinary volume that reflects the latest developments in autism spectrum disorder (ASD) research, practice, and theory. This collection brings together leading voices from biomedical science, behavioural psychology, neurodevelopmental research, and cognitive theory to explore how autism is understood, experienced, and supported across the lifespan.

Autism spectrum disorder is not a single condition with a single cause. It is a heterogeneous, multifaceted spectrum of developmental differences that impact communication, behaviour, sensory processing, and social engagement. As our understanding of autism has evolved, so too has our recognition of the many biological, psychological, and contextual factors that shape how individuals on the spectrum experience the world.

This volume is organized into two thematically distinct yet complementary sections. The first section, *Biological Foundations and Emerging Technologies in Autism Spectrum Disorders*, focuses on the physiological and technological aspects of autism. It includes an in-depth discussion of biomedical issues such as gut dysbiosis, nutritional deficiencies, and metabolic dysfunctions, highlighting their influence on mood, cognition, and daily functioning. Another chapter explores the promise of machine learning in early diagnosis, utilizing subtle motor patterns to detect signs of autism earlier and more objectively than traditional methods. This section also includes a review of genetic contributions to autism, particularly the role of copy number variations (CNVs), providing insights into how individual genetic profiles may influence the diverse expressions of ASD.

The second section, *Psychosocial Dynamics, Intervention Strategies, and Conceptual Perspectives in ASD*, turns toward the lived experience of autism and the human relationships that surround it. One chapter examines the benefits of parent-mediated interventions, providing both a practical framework and an overview of future directions in collaborative care. Another presents qualitative feedback from parents who participated in modified interaction therapy with their preschool children, capturing their emotional journeys, expectations, and transformative outcomes. Furthermore, this section reframes stereotypies and self-stimulatory behaviors not as pathological, but as meaningful self-regulation strategies that warrant understanding rather than suppression. The final chapter offers a bold conceptual exploration of autism, proposing the "Autistic Space Conjecture"—a philosophical and cognitive framework for understanding autistic consciousness and its distinct way of engaging with the world.

Together, these chapters offer a rich tapestry of perspectives—empirical, clinical, technological, and conceptual. While the contributors approach autism from different angles, a unifying theme emerges: autism must be understood in both its biological and behavioural dimensions, with attention to the whole person and their environment. There is no one-size-fits-all explanation or intervention. Instead, personalized approaches that draw from a range of disciplines and respect individual needs and neurodivergent identities are essential.

This book is designed for a broad audience. It will be valuable to researchers in neuroscience, psychology, and education, as well as to clinicians and therapists working in developmental and behavioural health, and to parents, caregivers, and self-advocates who seek a more comprehensive, evidence-based understanding of autism. It also serves as a resource for policymakers and educators seeking to align their efforts with the latest scientific and ethical thinking in the field.

*Bridging Biology and Behavior in Autism* encourages a shift in how we think about autism, from isolated symptoms to interconnected systems, from deficits to differences, and fixed diagnoses to evolving understandings. By integrating biological insight with behavioural expertise and lived experience, this volume contributes to a more compassionate, informed, and practical approach to supporting individuals on the autism spectrum throughout their lives.

**Marco Carotenuto**
Department of Mental and Physical Health and Preventive Medicine,
University of Campania "Luigi Vanvitelli",
Caserta, Italy

**Carola Costanza**
Department of Sciences for Health Promotion and Mother and Child Care
"G. D'Alessandro",
University of Palermo,
Palermo, Italy

Section 1

# Biological Foundations and Emerging Technologies in Autism Spectrum Disorders

**Chapter 1**

# Addressing Biomedical Issues, Including Gastrointestinal Issues, Gut Dysbiosis, Immune System Dysfunction, Nutritional Deficiencies, and Metabolic Imbalance in Autism Spectrum Disorder for a Healthier and Happier Outcome

*Joby Pulikkan, Deepa Azhchath Vasu, Mottakunja Deepthi and Tony Grace*

## Abstract

Autism spectrum disorder (ASD), with its increasing prevalence and lack of distinguished aetiology of pathogenesis, is, indeed, a topic worth in-depth research. This chapter explores the intricate interplay between gastrointestinal issues, gut dysbiosis, immune dysfunction, nutritional deficiencies, and metabolic imbalances in individuals with ASD. The complex bidirectional relationship between the gut and brain, often referred to as the gut-brain axis, plays a pivotal role in ASD. Gastrointestinal (GI) disturbances are prevalent in individuals with ASD, contributing to altered gut microbiota, a condition known as gut dysbiosis. This dysbiosis, in turn, can lead to an impaired immune system and chronic inflammation, further exacerbating behavioural and cognitive symptoms associated with ASD. This chapter delves into how gut dysbiosis impacts immune system function, highlighting the over-activation of the immune system and the production of pro-inflammatory cytokines. These immune alterations can create a cascade of effects, leading to nutritional deficiencies, particularly in essential vitamins and minerals. The body's ability to absorb and utilise these nutrients efficiently is compromised, which can affect metabolic processes and further contribute to the physiological and behavioural challenges observed in ASD. Furthermore, the chapter discusses briefly the potential therapeutic interventions aimed at restoring gut health, such as dietary modifications, probiotics, and prebiotics, which could alleviate some of the symptoms of ASD. By providing a comprehensive overview of the interconnected factors and their implications, this chapter underscores the importance of a holistic approach to understanding and managing ASD, considering the intricate relationships between the gut, immune system, nutrition, and metabolism.

**Keywords:** autism spectrum disorders, gastrointestinal issues, gut dysbiosis, microbial transplant therapy, dietary interventions

## 1. Introduction

Autism spectrum disorder is a debilitating neurodevelopmental disorder. Impaired social functioning and communication, repetitive behavioural patterns, and particular interests shown by the children with ASD prove that they have a variety of cognitive, social, behavioural, and health symptoms [1]. There are no reliable physiological markers for ASD to date. Currently, ASD is diagnosed by observing the patient in a set of social and behavioural tasks along with parental interviews under certain standardised behavioural scales [2]. The children with ASD show symptoms like hand flapping, walking on toes, refusal to eat, and staying awake all night [3]. Though ASD is a neurodevelopmental disorder, it is often misclassified as a psychiatric disorder due to its inclusion in the Diagnostic and Statistical Manual of Mental Disorders (DSM-5), leading to the oversight of biomedical issues that frequently co-occur with autism.

Biomedical issues, such as gastrointestinal problems, gut dysbiosis, immune system dysfunction, nutritional deficiencies and metabolic imbalance, are common in individuals with ASD. These comorbidities can significantly influence the health and well-being of individuals with ASD. Addressing these issues may be rewarding, as it leads to the alleviation of behavioural, cognitive and other allied psychiatric symptoms. The anecdotal experiences supported by evidence-based interventions from the physicians suggest that manipulating the biochemistry through diet and nutrition in children with autism is changing the course of the disease. The biochemistry of autism advocates that autism is much more than a developmental disorder, but it is, in fact, a complex metabolic disease affecting multiple organ systems.

## 2. Major biomedical issues found in autism spectrum disorder

### 2.1 Gastrointestinal issues and their impact on autism spectrum disorder

The inability of the medical establishment to look beyond the psychiatric model of autism has caused many of the physical symptoms common in patients with autism to largely go unrecognised or ignored. Recent medical literature clearly shows that gut symptoms are common in autism: Gastrointestinal (GI) symptoms are reported in 80% of the autistic population studies in Montreal [4]. A history of GI symptoms has been elicited in 70% of children with ASD compared with 28% of children with typical development and 42% of children with other developmental disabilities [5]. Similar rates are reported in various independent studies of American children with autism [6, 7]. It is suggested that symptoms such as unexplained irritability, aggressive behaviour, mood changes, discomfort, and nightmare awakenings could easily be dismissed or misinterpreted as neurological or "behavioural" rather than

*DOI: http://dx.doi.org/10.5772/intechopen.1010563*

manifestations of gastrointestinal discomfort in a nonverbal patient. Diagnostic confirmation of upper GI disease in autistic children was proven in a study by Horvath et al. [8]. The study cohort included children with autism and GI symptoms such as abdominal pain, chronic diarrhoea, gaseousness, bloating, night-time awakening, unexplained irritability and symptomatic food allergies. The study identified reflux oesophagitis, chronic stomach inflammation, inflammation in the duodenum and abnormal carbohydrate digestive enzymes in this study cohort. It has been furnished that ASD children, those with frequent abdominal pain, gaseousness, diarrhoea, constipation or pain on stooling, scored worse on irritability, social withdrawal, stereotypy and hyperactivity compared with children having no frequent GI symptoms [9]. Thus, it can be understood that maladaptive behaviours correlate with GI problems, suggesting these comorbidities require attention.

Among the GI problems recounted in subsets of autistic individuals, the most common are chronic constipation, diarrhoea and abdominal pain. Gastro-oesophageal reflux, bloody stools, vomiting and gaseousness are increasingly reported in some autistic individuals compared to their neurotypical counterparts. So are signs of GI inflammation, such as lymphoid nodular hyperplasia, complement activation, and elevated pro-inflammatory cytokines, and intestinal pathologies, such as enterocolitis, gastritis and oesophagitis [10, 11]. Increased intestinal permeability associated with autism is hypothesised to have harmful effects not just on intestinal barrier integrity [12], but further has a strong influence on the systemic metabolome, with possible translocation of intestinal metabolites or bacteria, thus promoting consequent immune activation [13]. Apart from the above-mentioned paraphernalia, food allergies, altered dietary nutrient intake and metabolic disruptions have been associated with ASD [14–16]. Altered carbohydrate digestion is also markedly reported in ASD individuals with comorbid GI abnormalities [17]. Thus, it is strongly suggested *via* the anecdotal reports and the extended research studies that the variety of GI conditions, dietary issues and enteric immune abnormalities reported in ASD individuals indicate that GI dysfunction can exacerbate the manifestation of core symptoms of autism. Several factors are believed to contribute to the GI issues in children, which include dietary habits, sensory sensitivities, behavioural factors, gut microbiota and genetic and environmental factors.

Selective eating, defined as restrictive eating behaviour with a limited number of preferred foods, is being considered as a nutritional problem in ASD. Since there is no consistent operational definition of selective eating, the prevalence of selective eating is difficult to estimate either in ASD or in children without ASD. But the current estimates suggest that selective eating is more prevalent in children with ASD than in typically developing children [18]. It is reported that food preferences, aversions, and refusal could be influenced by sensory sensitivity to textures, tastes, and smells in individuals with ASD [19]. It is also suggested that a high prevalence of co-occurring anxiety increases the risk of food neophobia, namely the fear of attempting new foods [20]. Studies have reported that children with ASD exhibited food selectivity towards starchy foods and consumed a smaller variety of foods compared to typically developing participants and often were reluctant to eat meat, eggs, rice, vegetables, and fruits [21]. Lower protein and calcium intake [22], prevalence of iron deficiency and anaemia [23] and significantly lower average levels of haemoglobin, ferritin, magnesium, potassium, calcium, phosphorus, glucose and haematocrit are also reported in autistic children [24]. Thus, it is evident that gastrointestinal issues found in ASD contribute to the exacerbation of ASD symptoms, and addressing these challenges can give a better outcome.

### 2.2 Unveiling the disrupted microbiome (gut dysbiosis) in autism spectrum disorder

The importance of gut microbiota for gastrointestinal functions is evident by their profound influence on both mucosal and systemic immunity. The emerging studies indicate that the microbiota significantly influences neurodevelopment and behaviour. Immune dysfunction and GI distress are extremely common in individuals with ASD, and a growing body of evidence suggests that gut dysbiosis could be exacerbating the ASD symptoms by its influence on immunity and metabolism. Though the pathogenesis of AD remains largely elusive, altered gut microbiome compositions leading to a situation called gut microbiome dysbiosis are very evident in ASD [25]. Common comorbidities like gastrointestinal symptoms and gut microbiome dysbiosis are presented to be correlated with the behavioural severity of ASD [26, 27].

Dysbiosis is known to promote activation of immune cells, including macrophages, which in turn produce quinolinic acid (QA). QA is a metabolite of the kynurenine pathway, which is involved in the metabolism of tryptophan. Elevated levels of QA have been associated with neuroinflammatory conditions and have been studied in relation to ASD. This metabolite has been correlated with the severity of certain diseases, including ASD [28]. Research suggests that QA may contribute to neuroinflammation and oxidative stress, which could potentially affect brain development and function in autistic children. However, more research is needed to fully understand its role and implications.

The characterisation of gut dysbiosis in ASD by various studies has indicated an increased amount of pathogenic bacteria and a reduced amount of beneficial bacteria. In metagenomics, alpha diversity characterises the richness and diversity of the microbiome in a solitary ecosystem. Operational taxonomic unit (OUT counts), Chaos 1 and Shannon index are the major alpha diversity metrics commonly used. No consistent patterns were available when it came to the study of alpha diversity on ASD. But beta diversity studies using Bray-Curtis dissimilarity, Jaccard distance, Unifrac, etc., which refer to the total variance in microbial community composition among the samples, reported significant differences in beta diversity. At the phylum level, the Firmicutes/Bacteroidetes ratio has been found disrupted in autistic subjects with a reduction in relative abundance of the Bacteroides phylum in ASD [29, 30]. At the genus level, studies have reported a decrease in the abundance of Alistipes, Bilophila, Dialister, Parabacteroides, Veillonella [30], Bacteroides, Bifidobacterium, Ruminococcus, Roseburia and Blautia [29] in children with ASD, while Collinsella, Corynebacterium, Dorea and Lactobacillus were significantly increased [30]. This study also made a very pivotal finding where they have identified that constipation is associated with different bacterial patterns in autistic children, as these children are characterised to have high levels of bacterial taxa belonging to Escherichia/Shigella and Clostridium cluster XVIII [30]. Current research studies also show elevated levels of pathogenic bacteria like Clostridium, Desulfovibrio, Proteobacteria, and Escherichia-Shigella in their gut microbiome [31–33] while showing reduced amounts of beneficial bacteria such as Bifidobacterium and Prevotella [34], exposing the potential link between gut dysbiosis and autism symptoms.

### 2.3 Immune system irregularities in ASD

Many studies over the last four decades have progressively recognised immune dysfunction in ASD as a significant factor contributing to the exacerbation of autistic symptoms. Strong inflammation states concomitant with ASD are often linked to immune system dysfunction [35, 36]. Pro-inflammatory biomarker analysis has revealed enhanced inflammatory activity in ASD children. Interleukins, known to be responsible for immune modulation and inflammatory responses, are considered optimal biomarkers for studying inflammatory responses [37]. Elevated pro-inflammatory cytokines such as IL-1β, IL-6, IL-8 and IL-12p40 have been reported in ASD compared with typically developing control children [38], suggesting that dysfunctional immune responses could affect core behaviours in autism. Alterations in immune cells such as T cells, B cells, monocytes, natural killer cells and dendritic cells have been reported in studies, along with alterations in immunoglobulins and autoantibodies. A great number of individuals with ASD are also reported to have elevated peripheral cytokines and chemokines, leading to neuroinflammation [39]. In a comprehensive assessment of the peripheral immune aberrations in subjects with ASD carried out in India, the researchers found no significant differences in the proportion of T regulatory cells, B cells, monocytes and natural killer cells between ASD subjects and controls. But the same study found the proportion of activated Th17 and myeloid dendritic cells significantly higher in children with ASD. Group comparison of serum levels of Th17 cytokines further revealed that serum levels of interleukin-17A were elevated, corroborating the immunophenotyping studies [40]. The role of this dysregulated pathway in the development of ASD assumes greater significance in the backdrop of a mice model study that had highlighted the role of the Th17 pathway in the pathophysiology of ASD [41]. Brain-specific autoantibodies and behaviour have been correlated in a large study involving 277 ASD children and 189 typically developing age-matched controls, which showed that children with the presence of autoantibodies showed lower adaptive and cognitive function while showing increased aberrant behaviours [42]. Immune system irregularities in ASD are manifested in various ways, including chronic inflammation, gut-brain axis, autoimmune responses, immunodeficiency, allergic reactions, etc.

### 2.4 Nutritional deficiencies in autism spectrum disorder

Nutritional health plays a crucial role in the overall well-being and development of children, yet children with autism spectrum disorder (ASD) often face unique dietary challenges that can lead to significant nutritional imbalances. Emerging research highlights a significant difference in the nutritional status of children with ASD compared to their typically developing peers [43]. Understanding these nutritional disparities is crucial in developing targeted interventions to improve dietary habits, optimise nutrient intake, and enhance overall well-being in individuals with autism. The several nutritional deficits that are frequently seen in ASD and their underlying causes are covered in this section of the review study.

According to research, children with ASD are five times more likely to experience eating disorders, which puts them at risk for nutritional deficiencies that could further affect their development, cognitive abilities and general health [44]. These eating disorders, often marked by selective food preferences, sensory sensitivities and gastrointestinal disturbances, can significantly limit nutrient intake, exacerbating the risk of deficiencies and their associated health impacts. Certain traits of ASD, including behavioural rigidity, a strong preference for routine and repetitive behaviours, can significantly influence food choices and eating patterns [45]. Children with ASD tend to have distinct sensory sensitivities, including heightened or diminished reactions to tactile, olfactory and visual stimuli that can contribute to rigid food preferences, often influenced by the food's texture, appearance, taste or temperature [46, 47]. These sensitivities frequently result in food neophobia, causing children to avoid certain foods and restrict their diet to a narrow range of selected foods that they consume consistently. Several studies of food consumption and nutritional intake in children with ASD have reported little variety in the diets of these children, a general preference for energy-dense foods, and a dislike for fruits, vegetables and dairy products [48, 49]. Children with ASD may also experience motor difficulties related to chewing and swallowing [50], as well as biological food intolerances or gastrointestinal issues [51]. The range of foods they can consume is further restricted by these considerations. Additionally, children with ASD often display challenging mealtime behaviours and are frequently perceived as "picky eaters" by their parents. They tend to exhibit strong food selectivity and pronounced dietary preferences, rejecting acidic foods and roughage while favouring sweet, energy-dense foods compared to their neurotypical peers [52]. These eating habits contribute to poor dietary patterns, characterised by a high intake of energy-dense snacks and ultra-processed foods coupled with a lower consumption of essential nutrients [53]. This imbalance can lead to nutrient deficiencies and related health complications. Moreover, gastrointestinal issues are common in autism and can disrupt the absorption of essential nutrients, leading to nutritional deficiencies [54]. Conditions such as diarrhoea, constipation, abdominal discomfort and gastric acid imbalances are frequently observed in children with ASD and may reduce the absorption of essential nutrients [55].

Given the nutritional imbalance observed in children with ASD compared to typically developing children, it is essential to identify the specific nutrients that are deficient. Recent studies have identified deficiencies in several nutrients, including vitamins (A, D, C, B1, B2, B5, B6, B9, and B12) [44, 56, 57], omega-3 fatty acids (docosahexaenoic acid and docosapentaenoic acid) [58, 59] and macrominerals (calcium, iron, phosphorus, selenium and zinc) [43, 57, 60] in children with ASD. Research has highlighted insufficient intake of vitamin A (β-carotene and retinol) in children with ASD, a micronutrient crucial for growth, vision and central nervous system function. Guo et al. [61] reported that such deficiencies may not only disrupt these fundamental physiological processes but also aggravate ASD-related symptoms and behavioural disturbances. Vitamin D deficiency is associated with hypocalcaemia, which can negatively impact bone mass development. This effect may be more pronounced in children with ASD, as reviewed by Abadi et al. [62], who reported lower bone density in children with ASD compared to their typically developing peers. Vitamin C plays a vital role in human health by supporting immune function, acting as a powerful antioxidant, promoting collagen synthesis for skin and tissue repair, enhancing iron absorption and contributing to overall cellular protection and metabolic processes [63]. Vitamin C deficiency in children with autism spectrum disorder (ASD) can lead to scurvy, presenting with symptoms such as musculoskeletal pain and fatigue, which may exacerbate behavioural challenges. A case report by Sakamornchai et al. [64] highlighted instances where children with ASD and vitamin C deficiency developed pulmonary arterial hypertension, underscoring the critical importance of adequate vitamin C intake in this population. Similarly, deficiencies in B-complex vitamins, including B6, B12 and folate, have been linked to neurological impairments and behavioural challenges in children with ASD [65]. Studies suggest that inadequate levels of these vitamins may contribute to increased oxidative stress, impaired methylation processes and neurotransmitter imbalances, potentially exacerbating ASD symptoms [66]. Through examining plasma profiles, urine samples and dietary intake, researchers found that abnormal amino acid and low B vitamin levels were present in children with ASD compared to those without ASD [67].

Omega-3 fatty acids play a crucial role in neurodevelopment, neurotransmission and synaptic plasticity, making their deficiency particularly concerning in ASD [68]. Emerging evidence suggests that inadequate levels of omega-3 fatty acids, particularly docosahexaenoic acid (DHA) and eicosapentaenoic acid (EPA), may exacerbate ASD symptoms by impairing cognitive function, increasing neuroinflammation and disrupting neuronal connectivity [69]. Moreover, omega-3 fatty acids are essential for modulating dopamine and serotonin pathways, both of which are implicated in ASD pathophysiology [70]. Studies have shown that omega-3 supplementation can improve attention, reduce hyperactivity and enhance social interactions in children with ASD, highlighting the critical role of these essential fatty acids in mitigating the disorder's severity [59].

Mineral deficiencies are increasingly recognised as a contributing factor to the severity of autism spectrum disorder (ASD), given their essential roles in neurodevelopment, neurotransmission and metabolic processes [71]. Children with ASD often exhibit deficiencies in key minerals such as zinc, magnesium, calcium and iron, which may exacerbate core symptoms of the disorder [72]. Zinc is crucial for synaptic function, immune regulation and antioxidant defence, and its deficiency has been associated with increased oxidative stress, impaired neuroplasticity and worsened behavioural symptoms in ASD [60, 73]. Magnesium plays a vital role in regulating neurotransmitter activity and neuronal excitability, and inadequate levels have been linked to heightened irritability, excitability and noise disturbance that could exacerbate ASD symptoms [74]. Related to vitamin D, Arija et al. [44] reported a highly inadequate intake of calcium in ASD children, which may also have an adverse effect on bone health. Low levels of calcium can increase the risk of osteomalacia and osteoporosis due to its important role in bone osteogenesis during childhood [75]. Guo et al. [76] suggested that calcium deficiency may be linked to the severity of social impairment in children with ASD [77]. Furthermore, adequate levels of calcium and iron have been associated with optimal cognitive and neurological function in children with ASD, emphasising the crucial role of these nutrients in shaping the social behaviours observed in individuals with ASD [44]. Additionally, iron is critical for dopamine synthesis and myelination, and its deficiency has been correlated with cognitive impairments, attention deficits and increased irritability in ASD [23]. Addressing these mineral deficiencies through targeted nutritional interventions may help mitigate some of the neurological and behavioural challenges associated with ASD. As essential structural and functional components of the central nervous system, micronutrients play a crucial role in the formation and regulation of the central nervous system and are essential to many physiological processes. Micronutrients also promote the migration, differentiation and growth of nerve cells. Consequently, deficiencies in micronutrients are anticipated to have a profound effect on both cognitive function and physical health in children with ASD [78].

In conclusion, assessing the dietary needs of children with ASD is crucial to prevent nutrient deficiencies through appropriate dietary modifications or supplementation with essential vitamins and minerals. Furthermore, research by Moiniafshari et al. [79] highlights that integrating nutrition and exercise programmes can have a more substantial positive impact on individuals with ASD when implemented together, emphasising the need for a comprehensive approach to improving their overall health and well-being.

## 2.5 Metabolic disorders found in autism

The diverse etiopathological landscape of ASD presents a broad and heterogeneous display that includes a wide range of cognitive, behavioural and sensory impairments. This heterogeneity suggests a complex interplay of genetic, environmental and metabolic factors underlying ASD pathophysiology [80].

Emerging evidence suggests that metabolic dysfunction plays a crucial role in ASD, contributing to neurodevelopmental abnormalities and symptom severity. Several metabolic pathways, including mitochondrial function, oxidative stress regulation, gastrointestinal disturbances and neurotransmitter metabolism, are frequently disrupted in individuals with ASD [81]. Additionally, methylation processes, impaired glucose metabolism and lipid imbalances further highlight the systemic nature of metabolic abnormalities in ASD. Understanding these metabolic disruptions may offer insights into potential biomarkers and therapeutic targets for ASD management.

Various inborn errors of metabolism have been identified in a subset of individuals with ASD, which includes mitochondrial dysfunction, oxidative stress and redox imbalances, being among the most frequently observed. Additionally, disruptions in methylation and folate metabolism, aberrant amino acid and neurotransmitter pathways, and gastrointestinal and microbiome dysregulation, as well as impairments in carbohydrate, lipid and cholesterol metabolism, have been implicated in ASD pathophysiology [82]. Since metabolic disorders are multisystemic, they attract involvement in various organ ailments and dysfunctions, which explains the factors contributing to the classic comorbid phenotypes found in ASD [83].

Mitochondrial dysfunction is often noted among ASD patients, impacting the vital energy-generating organelles referred to as the "powerhouses of the cell." Dysfunction can be caused by mutations in mtDNA or modified by exogenous and endogenous risk factors, resulting in structural and functional mitochondrial dysfunction [84]. Due to their pivotal function in cellular metabolism, mitochondria directly influence ASD pathophysiology as the key site of production of adenosine triphosphate (ATP), the fuel for regular brain function and synaptic transmission. Additionally, mitochondria control neurotransmitter function and cell homeostasis by controlling the levels of reactive oxygen species (ROS) and reactive nitrogen species (RNS) that are essential in physiological processes [85]. Multiple studies have revealed associations between mitochondrial dysfunction and ASD, and most ASD children had pronounced mitochondrial biomarker abnormalities in plasma lactate, ubiquinone, acyl-carnitine, and pyruvate concentrations and increased lactate-to-pyruvate and alanine-to-lysine ratios, again testifying to the participation of mitochondrial abnormalities in the development of ASD [86–88]. Genetic causes also underlie mitochondrial dysfunction in ASD. Genes such as SLC25A12, TMLHE and IMMP2L are autism-risk genes, and they have an important role in mitochondrial function, such as energy metabolism, fatty acid transport and regulation of oxidative stress [89]. These results point to mitochondrial dysfunction as one of the major factors in the multifactorial aetiology of ASD.

Recent studies have established a strong association between ASD and elevated oxidative stress, along with abnormalities in redox metabolism, suggesting their potential role in ASD pathogenesis [90, 91]. Oxidative stress contributes to ASD through multiple mechanisms, including protein carbonylation, disrupted metabolic pathways and the accumulation of reactive oxygen species (ROS) [92].

The interaction of genetic and environmental factors in individuals with ASD leads to excessive ROS production, reduced antioxidant defences and mitochondrial dysfunction, all of which collectively exacerbate oxidative stress. This oxidative imbalance can induce epigenetic dysregulation, neurodevelopmental abnormalities, neuroinflammation, cerebral injury and neuronal dysfunction, ultimately contributing to ASD development. Potential oxidative stress biomarkers associated with ASD have been identified, including blood- and urine-based markers such as glutathione, homocysteine, B vitamins, malondialdehyde (MDA) and 4-hydroxynonenal, all of which show significantly altered levels in individuals with ASD [93]. Glutathione metabolism plays a critical role in ASD pathophysiology through its regulation of redox homeostasis and redox-independent mechanisms. Key plasma markers of redox metabolism include reduced free glutathione (fGSH), oxidised glutathione (GSSG), the fGSH/GSSG ratio and 3-nitrotyrosine (3NT) [94]. Moreover, mitochondrial dysfunction and neuronal apoptosis are pivotal links between impaired glutathione metabolism and ASD, highlighting the interconnected roles of oxidative stress, redox imbalance and mitochondrial abnormalities in the disorder's pathogenesis [95].

Scientific evidence indicates that children with ASD can have compromised methylation and folate metabolism. Research shows that disturbed methylation, along with enhanced oxidative stress, is responsible for the pathophysiology of ASD [96–98]. The methionine cycle, which is essential for fundamental cellular processes, is vital in the methylation of DNA, RNA, proteins and other molecules. The decline in methionine concentration because of impaired methylation has been linked to enhanced oxidative stress in ASD populations [99]. Likewise, folate, which is required for DNA synthesis *via* purine and pyrimidine biosynthesis, is critical in ensuring cellular processes. Abnormalities and impairments in the methionine cycle, frequently due to folate metabolism or transport abnormalities, have been implicated in the pathogenesis of ASD [100, 101]. Research has shown the interdependence between reduced folate levels and disturbed methylation among autistic children to result in metabolic changes related to learning disabilities, behavioural problems and neuropsychological impairments [102–104].

Dysregulations of amino acid and neurotransmitter metabolism have been implicated increasingly in the pathophysiology underlying the cognitive, behavioural and various neurodevelopmental manifestations observed in ASD [105–107]. Studies in children with ASD have reported altered levels of amino acids, including phenylalanine (Phe), glutamine (Gln), glycine (Gly), leucine (Leu), arginine (Arg), lysine (Lys), serine (Ser), taurine (Tau), tryptophan (Trp), threonine (Thr), methionine (Met) and histidine (His) in serum and plasma [108–110]. These amino acids play essential roles in cellular function, immune regulation, metabolism and neurotransmission, and their dysregulation is associated with metabolic abnormalities observed in ASD. Excitatory and inhibitory neurotransmissions, the main mediators of which are glutamate and gamma-aminobutyric acid (GABA), have an important role in regulating normal brain function [111]. A persistent imbalance marked by increased glutamate and decreased GABAergic signalling changes has been consistently observed in ASD individuals [112]. Such excitatory-inhibitory dysregulation can give rise to hyperexcitability of neural circuits, manifesting heightened anxiety, sensory hypersensitivity and social communication impairment. Additionally, genetic mutations involving glutamate receptors as well as GABAergic signalling pathways highlight their role in ASD pathogenesis [113]. Two neurotransmitters, serotonin and dopamine, involved in mood regulation, behaviour and cognitive processes, were also found dysregulated in ASD [114, 115]. A disrupted serotonin metabolism, particularly hyperserotonemia (elevated whole-blood serotonin concentrations), was reported in a clinically relevant subgroup of patients with ASD. This serotonergic dysregulation was linked to stereotypies, communication deficits and gastrointestinal disturbances associated with ASD [116]. Similarly, observations in dopamine signalling pathways were associated with attention deficits, reward inhibition and motor control problems [35]. Studies reported the genetic variations of several dopaminergic genes, such as the genes-encoding dopamine receptors and transporters, revealing the heritability of dopaminergic dysfunction in ASD [117].

Amino acid metabolism and neurotransmitter system dysregulation have a remarkable influence on cognitive functions and behavioural phenotypes in ASD. Synaptic plasticity is prone to be impeded by this excitatory-inhibitory imbalance, which potentially disturbs learning and memory processes. Moreover, serotonergic and dopaminergic abnormalities contribute to mood disorders, attentional deficits, repetitive behaviours and deficits in social communication. Such neurochemical alterations may contribute to the diverse phenotypic features of ASD and add layers of complexity to the biochemical basis underlying these disorders, revealing areas for potential therapeutic manipulations through neurotransmitter/peptide systems that may mitigate cognitive or behaviour-related anomalies associated with ASD.

Gastrointestinal (GI) distress is frequently reported in those with ASD, commonly visualised as constipation, diarrhoea, discomfort of the abdomen and bloating [118, 119]. Newly available data indicate that these GI symptoms are closely associated with changes in the gut microbiome, which plays an important role in brain function and behaviour *via* the gut-brain axis [120]. It has been suggested that dysregulation of a bidirectional network of the gut-brain axis, rather than the other, which is related to gastrointestinal tract function, is involved in gastrointestinal issues with neurobehavioural symptoms in ASD [121]. Changes in gut permeability (known as leaky gut), immune activation and changes in gut-generated metabolites, in particular, may alter neurodevelopment, synaptic plasticity and neurotransmission and may potentiate symptoms consistent with ASD, including irritability, anxiety and social interactions [122].

Individuals with ASD have a significantly different microbiome composition than neurotypical controls, with a distinct decrease in microbial diversity and an alteration of specific bacterial taxa [123, 124]. Studies have uniformly reported higher abundances of *Clostridium*, *Esulfovibrio*, *Sutterella* and *Bacteroides* species and lower levels of beneficial commensals like *Bifidobacterium* [125, 126]. These microbial imbalances can interfere with the production of vital microbial metabolites, provoke immune dysregulation and promote gastrointestinal inflammation, all of which may contribute to ASD pathophysiology [127].

Short-chain fatty acids (SCFAs), such as acetate, propionate and butyrate, are key microbiota-derived metabolites stemming from the fermentation of dietary fibres in the gut. SCFAs can act as important contributors for preserving intestinal permeability, regulating the immune system and affecting central nervous system actions [128–130]. In ASD, aberrant SCFA profiles, especially increased propionic acid levels, have been linked to neuroinflammation, mitochondrial abnormalities and altered neurotransmitter systems [131, 132]. The association between propionic acid and ASD has been supported by experimental models where excessive propionic acid exposure would induce ASD-like behavioural phenotypes, thereby implicating propionic acid as a potential contributor to ASD pathogenesis [133].

Emerging research suggests that disruptions in carbohydrate metabolism may contribute to the pathogenesis of ASD and influence its clinical implications [17]. One key aspect of carbohydrate metabolism dysregulation in ASD is insulin resistance, a condition in which cells fail to respond adequately to insulin, which has been reported in some individuals with ASD and may be linked to the development of metabolic disorders that are more common in this population. Glucose, the primary energy source for the brain, is critical for neurodevelopment, synaptic function and neurotransmission. Impaired glucose metabolism, including insulin resistance and dysfunctional glucose transport, has been increasingly associated with ASD-related neurodevelopmental abnormalities [134].

Insulin has an important role in modulating neuronal growth, synaptic plasticity and cognitive function. Disruption of insulin signalling in ASD has been shown to contribute to metabolic and neurological impairment. Individuals with ASD have been found to have an increased rate of insulin resistance and metabolic syndrome, implicating a potential metabolic basis for the disorder [135]. Insulin resistance can result in decreased neuronal glucose uptake, disrupting energy production and synaptic function, thus contributing to cognitive and behavioural impairments in ASD [136]. Insulin resistance is usually associated with mitochondrial dysfunction, resulting in enhanced oxidative stress and disrupted neuronal energy metabolism, both of which are commonly observed in ASD. One of the most important features of carbohydrate metabolism dysregulation in ASD is insulin resistance, a state where cells do not respond to insulin, the hormone that regulates blood glucose levels, appropriately. Insulin resistance has been described in some with ASD and could be associated with the development of more prevalent metabolic disorders, including type 2 diabetes, in this group [137, 138].

In addition, impairments in glucose transport, or the mechanism through which glucose is brought to cells for energy metabolism, have been seen in ASD as well. Adequate glucose transport through the blood-brain barrier is required for neuronal health and neurodevelopmental support [139]. Abnormality in the dysregulation of glucose transporter proteins has been noted in ASD, further implicating metabolic dysregulation in its pathophysiology [140]. Impaired expression of glucose transporter proteins such as GLUT1, GLUT3 and GLUT4, can be a cause of altered neuronal glucose uptake, resulting in impaired synaptic plasticity, neurotransmitter synthesis and neuronal connectivity [141–144]. Neuroimaging studies employing fluorodeoxyglucose positron emission tomography have shown decreased cerebral glucose metabolism in patients with ASD, especially in areas related to social cognition, executive function and communication [145]. Chronic disturbances of glucose metabolism could impair early brain development, myelination and neuronal differentiation, leading to the cognitive and behavioural phenotypes of ASD [146].

Similarly, lipid metabolism and cholesterol imbalances have been involved in the aetiopathology of ASD, with many studies emphasising their role in neurodevelopment [147, 148]. Lipids and cholesterol are ubiquitous constituents of the brain, which play crucial functions in myelin sheaths, neuronal membranes, astrocytes and grey matter. They play vital roles in preserving the intricate morphology of the neurons and aiding synaptic transmission. In contrast to peripheral cholesterol, which is systemically synthesised, brain cholesterol is locally produced, hence a prime area of study in ASD. Disturbances in cholesterol homeostasis have been shown to directly influence synaptic transmission, ultimately compromising brain function and the manifestation of cognitive and behavioural manifestations in ASD [149]. Dysregulated lipid metabolism not only disrupts myelination and neurotransmitter transport but also facilitates neuroinflammation, all of which are essential for normal brain development and function [150]. Altered membrane fluidity, defective synaptic transmission and disrupted neuronal connectivity have been reported in ASD, possibly associated with lipid metabolism abnormalities. Several studies have reported genetic and metabolic abnormalities in lipid pathways, such as mutations in genes responsible for lipid transport and synthesis [151]. In addition to their morphological functions, lipids play key roles in neuronal signalling, synaptic plasticity, release of neurotransmitters and calcium signalling [152]. Some of the evidence that suggests the role of lipid dysregulation in ASD includes changed levels of cholesterol, abnormal ganglioside composition and distinctive metabolic patterns reported in affected individuals.

## 3. Potential therapeutic interventions in ASD by addressing the biomedical issues

A range of interventions aimed at targeting underlying physiological and biochemical imbalances are attempted, which are briefly described here.

### 3.1 Addressing gut health using probiotics, prebiotics and synbiotics

Probiotics, prebiotics and synbiotics can help restore gut health and reduce gastrointestinal issues. Probiotics are beneficial bacteria, while prebiotics are those that promote the growth of healthy gut bacteria. Synbiotics are the prebiotics and probiotics.

### 3.2 Addressing gut health using microbial transplant therapy

Dr. James B Adams has conducted research on the use of Microbiota Transplant Therapy (MTT), a special type of faecal transplant, to treat ASD symptoms. This therapy involves transferring gut microbiota from healthy donors to individuals with ASD, aiming to restore a healthy gut microbiome. Studies show that MTT can lead to significant improvements in gut health and a reduction in ASD symptoms [153].

### 3.3 Dietary interventions for a healthier outcome in ASD

Gluten-free and casein-free (GCFC) Diets: These diets eliminate gluten and casein, which are thought to exacerbate ASD symptoms in some individuals. Specific carbohydrate diet (SCD): This diet focuses on removing complex carbohydrates to improve gut health [154].

### 3.4 Nutritional supplements to address deficiencies in ASD

Omega-3 fatty acids are believed to enhance brain function and reduce inflammation. Adequate levels of vitamin D are essential for immune function and overall health. Antioxidant supplements such as coenzyme Q10 and N-acetyl cysteine can help reduce oxidative stress. Nutrients like carnitine can support mitochondrial function. Melatonin, vitamin C, krill oil, fish oil, vitamin D, magnesium, Epsom salts and zinc are also found to be beneficial for addressing ASD-related symptoms [155].

## 4. Conclusion

To conclude, this chapter review titled "Addressing Biomedical Issues, Including Gastrointestinal Issues, Gut Dysbiosis, Immune System Dysfunction, Nutritional Deficiencies, and Metabolic Imbalance in Autism Spectrum Disorder for a Healthier and Happier Outcome," underscores the critical role of biomedical interventions in improving the quality of life for individuals with ASD. This chapter tries to provide a comprehensive understanding of the multifaceted nature of ASD by exploring the intricate interplay between gastrointestinal health, gut microbiota, immune function, nutritional status and metabolic processes. This review highlights the importance of considering biomedical issues in the efficient management of ASD. Interventions such as dietary modifications, nutritional supplementation and therapies aimed at restoring gut health have shown promising results in alleviating symptoms and improving overall well-being. The chapter also emphasises the need for personalised treatment plans, as each individual with ASD presents unique challenges and requires tailored interventions. Navigating through current research and clinical practices, this chapter provides valuable insights into the potential benefits of addressing biomedical issues in ASD. By adopting a multi-tiered approach and integrating biomedical interventions with behavioural therapies, one can pave the way for healthier and happier outcomes for individuals with ASD and their families.

## Acknowledgements

The authors acknowledge the usage of QuillBot, Copilot and ChatGPT (AI tools used) for language polishing and paraphrasing of the manuscript.

## Author details

Joby Pulikkan[1*], Deepa Azhchath Vasu[2], Mottakunja Deepthi[2] and Tony Grace[2]

1 St. John's National Academy of Health Sciences, St. John's Research Institute, Bangalore, India

2 Department of Genomic Science, School of Biological Sciences, Central University of Kerala, India

*Address all correspondence to: puljobcmi@gmail.com

## References

[1] Osredkar J, Baškovič BŽ, Finderle P, Bobrowska-Korczak B, Gątarek P, Rosiak A, et al. Relationship between excreted uremic toxins and degree of disorder of children with ASD. International Journal of Molecular Sciences. 2023;**24**(8):7078

[2] Olesova D, Galba J, Piestansky J, Celusakova H, Repiska G, Babinska K, et al. A novel UHPLC-MS method targeting urinary metabolomic markers for autism spectrum disorder. Metabolites. 2020;**10**(11):443

[3] Signs and Symptoms of Autism Spectrum Disorder. Available from: https://www.cdc.gov/autism/signs-symptoms/index.html

[4] D'Souza Y, Fombonne E, Ward BJ. No evidence of persisting measles virus in peripheral blood mononuclear cells from children with autism spectrum disorder. Pediatrics. 2006;**118**(4):1664-1675

[5] Valicenti-McDermott M, McVicar KA, Rapin I, Wershil BK, Cohen H, Shinnar S. Frequency of gastrointestinal symptoms in children with autistic spectrum disorders and association with family history of autoimmune disease. Journal of Developmental and Behavioral Pediatrics. 2006;**27**(2):S128-S136

[6] Melmed RD, Schneider C, Fabes R, Philips J, Reichelt K. Metabolic markers and gastrointestinal symptoms in children with autism and related disorders. Journal of Pediatric Gastroenterology and Nutrition. 2000;**31**(Suppl. 2):S31

[7] Horvath K, Perman JA. Autistic disorder and gastrointestinal disease. Current Opinion in Pediatrics. 2002;**14**(5):583-587

[8] Horvath K, Papadimitriou JC, Rabsztyn A, Drachenberg C, Tildon JT. Gastrointestinal abnormalities in children with autistic disorder. The Journal of Pediatrics. 1999;**135**(5):559-563

[9] Chaidez V, Hansen RL, Hertz-Picciotto I. Gastrointestinal problems in children with autism, developmental delays or typical development. Journal of Autism and Developmental Disorders. 2014;**44**:1117-1127

[10] Buie T, Campbell DB, Fuchs GJ III, Furuta GT, Levy J, Vandewater J, et al. Evaluation, diagnosis, and treatment of gastrointestinal disorders in individuals with ASDs: A consensus report. Pediatrics. 2010;**125**(Suppl. 1):S1-S8

[11] Coury DL, Ashwood P, Fasano A, Fuchs G, Geraghty M, Kaul A, et al. Gastrointestinal conditions in children with autism spectrum disorder: Developing a research agenda. Pediatrics. 2012;**130**(Suppl. 2):S160-S168

[12] De Magistris L, Familiari V, Pascotto A, Sapone A, Frolli A, Iardino P, et al. Alterations of the intestinal barrier in patients with autism spectrum disorders and in their first-degree relatives. Journal of Pediatrics Gastroenterology and Nutrition. 2010;**51**(4):418-424

[13] Erickson CA, Stigler KA, Corkins MR, Posey DJ, Fitzgerald JF, McDougle CJ. Gastrointestinal factors in autistic disorder: A critical review. Journal of Autism and Developmental Disorders. 2005;**35**:713-727

[14] Levy SE, Souders MC, Ittenbach RF, Giarelli E, Mulberg AE, Pinto-Martin JA. Relationship of dietary intake to gastrointestinal symptoms in children

with autistic spectrum disorders. Biological Psychiatry. 2007;**61**(4):492-497

[15] Jyonouchi H. Food allergy and autism spectrum disorders: Is there a link? Current Allergy and Asthma Reports. 2009;**9**(3):194-201

[16] Ming X, Stein TP, Barnes V, Rhodes N, Guo L. Metabolic perturbance in autism spectrum disorders: A metabolomics study. Journal of Proteome Research. 2012;**11**:5856-5862

[17] Williams BL, Hornig M, Buie T, Bauman ML, Cho Paik M, Wick I, et al. Impaired carbohydrate digestion and transport and mucosal dysbiosis in the intestines of children with autism and gastrointestinal disturbances. PLoS ONE. 2011;**6**(9):e24585

[18] Önal S, Sachadyn-Król M, Kostecka M. A review of the nutritional approach and the role of dietary components in children with autism spectrum disorders in light of the latest scientific research. Nutrients. 2023;**15**(23):4852

[19] Johnson CR, Turner K, Stewart PA, Schmidt B, Shui A, Macklin E, et al. Relationships between feeding problems, behavioral characteristics and nutritional quality in children with ASD. Journal of Autism and Developmental Disorders. 2014;**44**:2175-2184

[20] Ung D, Selles R, Small BJ, Storch EA. A systematic review and meta-analysis of cognitive-behavioral therapy for anxiety in youth with high-functioning autism spectrum disorders. Child Psychiatry and Human Development. 2015;**46**:533-547

[21] Leila Cherif JB, Khemekhem K, Mkawer S, Ayadi H, Moalla Y. Feeding problems in children with autism spectrum disorders. Journal of Family Medicine. 2020;**1**:30-39

[22] Sharp WG, Postorino V, McCracken CE, Berry RC, Criado KK, Burrell TL, et al. Dietary intake, nutrient status, and growth parameters in children with autism spectrum disorder and severe food selectivity: An electronic medical record review. Journal of the Academy of Nutrition and Dietetics. 2018;**118**(10):1943-1950

[23] Pivina L, Semenova Y, Doşa MD, Dauletyarova M, Bjørklund G. Iron deficiency, cognitive functions, and neurobehavioral disorders in children. Journal of Molecular Neuroscience. 2019;**68**:1-10

[24] Bener A, Khattab AO, Bhugra D, Hoffmann GF. Iron and vitamin D levels among autism spectrum disorders children. Annals of African Medicine. 2017;**16**:186-191

[25] Pulikkan J, Maji A, Dhakan DB, Saxena R, Mohan B, Anto MM, et al. Gut microbial dysbiosis in Indian children with autism spectrum disorders. Microbial Ecology. 2018;**76**:1102-1114

[26] Wasilewska J, Klukowski M. Gastrointestinal symptoms and autism spectrum disorder: Links and risks–a possible new overlap syndrome. Pediatric Health, Medicine and Therapeutics. 2015;**6**:153-166

[27] Fattorusso A, Di Genova L, Dell'Isola GB, Mencaroni E, Esposito S. Autism spectrum disorders and the gut microbiota. Nutrients. 2019;**11**(3):521

[28] Saade MC, Clark AJ, Parikh SM. States of quinolinic acid excess in urine: A systematic review of human studies. Frontiers in Nutrition. 2022;**9**:1070435

[29] Niu M, Li Q, Zhang J, Wen F, Dang W, Duan G, et al. Characterization of intestinal microbiota and probiotics treatment in children with autism

spectrum disorders in China. Frontiers in Neurology. 2019;**10**:1084

[30] Strati F, Cavalieri D, Albanese D, De Felice C, Donati C, Hayek J, et al. New evidences on the altered gut microbiota in autism spectrum disorders. Microbiome. 2017;**5**:1-1

[31] Xu M, Xu X, Li J, Li F. Association between gut microbiota and autism spectrum disorder: A systematic review and meta-analysis. Frontiers in Psychiatry. 2019;**10**:473

[32] Karnachuk OV, Ikkert OP, Avakyan MR, Knyazev YV, Volochaev MN, Zyusman VS, et al. Desulfovibrio desulfuricans AY5 isolated from a patient with autism spectrum disorder binds iron in low-soluble greigite and pyrite. Microorganisms. 2021;**9**(12):2558

[33] Shin NR, Whon TW, Bae JW. Proteobacteria: Microbial signature of dysbiosis in gut microbiota. Trends in Biotechnology. 2015;**33**(9):496-503

[34] Kang DW, Park JG, Ilhan ZE, Wallstrom G, LaBaer J, Adams JB, et al. Reduced incidence of Prevotella and other fermenters in intestinal microflora of autistic children. PLoS ONE. 2013;**8**(7):e68322

[35] Croonenberghs J, Bosmans E, Deboutte D, Kenis G, Maes M. Activation of the inflammatory response system in autism. Neuropsychobiology. 2002;**45**(1):1-6

[36] Siniscalco D, Schultz S, Brigida AL, Antonucci N. Inflammation and neuro-immune dysregulations in autism spectrum disorders. Pharmaceuticals. 2018;**11**(2):56

[37] Brocker C, Thompson D, Matsumoto A, Nebert DW, Vasiliou V. Evolutionary divergence and functions of the human interleukin (IL) gene family. Human Genomics. 2010;**5**:1-26

[38] Ashwood P, Krakowiak P, Hertz-Picciotto I, Hansen R, Pessah I, Van de Water J. Elevated plasma cytokines in autism spectrum disorders provide evidence of immune dysfunction and are associated with impaired behavioral outcome. Brain, Behavior, and Immunity. 2011;**25**(1):40-45

[39] Bjorklund G, Saad K, Chirumbolo S, Kern J, Geier D, Geier M, et al. Immune dysfunction and neuroinflammation in autism spectrum disorder. Acta Neurobiologiae Experimentalis. 2016;**76**(4):257-268

[40] Basheer S, Venkataswamy MM, Christopher R, Van Amelsvoort T, Srinath S, Girimaji SC, et al. Immune aberrations in children with autism spectrum disorder: A case-control study from a tertiary care neuropsychiatric hospital in India. Psychoneuroendocrinology. 2018;**94**:162-167

[41] Choi GB, Yim YS, Wong H, Kim S, Kim H, Kim SV, et al. The maternal interleukin-17a pathway in mice promotes autism-like phenotypes in offspring. Science. 2016;**351**(6276):933-939

[42] Goines P, Haapanen L, Boyce R, Duncanson P, Braunschweig D, Delwiche L, et al. Autoantibodies to cerebellum in children with autism associate with behavior. Brain, Behavior, and Immunity. 2011;**25**(3):514-523

[43] Długosz A, Wróblewski M, Błaszak B, Szulc J. The role of nutrition, oxidative stress, and trace elements in the pathophysiology of autism spectrum disorders. International Journal of Molecular Sciences. 2025;**26**(2):808

[44] Arija V, Esteban-Figuerola P, Morales-Hidalgo P, Jardí C, Canals-Sans J. Nutrient intake and adequacy in children with autism spectrum disorder: EPINED epidemiological study. Autism. 2023;**27**(2):371-388

[45] Lung SL, Picard È, Soulières I, Bertone A. Identifying the functions of restricted and repetitive behaviours and interests in autism: A scoping review. Research in Autism Spectrum Disorders. 2024;**117**:102458

[46] Esposito M, Mirizzi P, Fadda R, Pirollo C, Ricciardi O, Mazza M, et al. Food selectivity in children with autism: Guidelines for assessment and clinical interventions. International Journal of Environmental Research and Public Health. 2023;**20**(6):5092

[47] Calisan Kinter R, Ozbaran B, Inal Kaleli I, Kose S, Bildik T, Ghaziuddin M. The sensory profiles, eating behaviors, and quality of life of children with autism spectrum disorder and avoidant/restrictive food intake disorder. Psychiatric Quarterly. 2024;**95**(1):85-106

[48] Canals-Sans J, Esteban-Figuerola P, Morales-Hidalgo P, Arija V. Do children with autism spectrum disorders eat differently and less adequately than those with subclinical ASD and typical development? EPINED epidemiological study. Journal of Autism and Developmental Disorders. 2022;**52**(1):361-375

[49] Esteban-Figuerola P, Canals J, Fernández-Cao JC, Arija VV. Differences in food consumption and nutritional intake between children with autism spectrum disorders and typically developing children: A meta-analysis. Autism. 2019;**23**(5):1079-1095

[50] Cerchiari A, Giordani C, Franceschetti S, Mazzafoglia S, Carosi F, Pizza F, et al. The efficacy of the global intensive feeding therapy on feeding and swallowing abilities in children with autism spectrum disorder: A pilot study. Children. 2023;**10**(7):1241

[51] Rodop BB, Başkaya E, Altuntaş İ, Erbaş O. Nutrition effect on autism spectrum disorders. Journal of Experimental and Basic Medical Sciences. 2021;**2**(1):007-017

[52] Leader G, Tuohy E, Chen JL, Mannion A, Gilroy SP. Feeding problems, gastrointestinal symptoms, challenging behavior and sensory issues in children and adolescents with autism spectrum disorder. Journal of Autism and Developmental Disorders. 2020;**50**:1401-1410

[53] Plaza-Diaz J, Flores-Rojas K, Torre-Aguilar MJ, Gomez-Fernández AR, Martín-Borreguero P, Perez-Navero JL, et al. Dietary patterns, eating behavior, and nutrient intakes of spanish preschool children with autism spectrum disorders. Nutrients. 2021;**13**(10):3551

[54] Almohmadi NH. Brain-gut-brain axis, nutrition, and autism spectrum disorders: A review. Translational Pediatrics. 2024;**13**(9):1652

[55] Al-Beltagi M, Saeed NK, Bediwy AS, Elbeltagi R, Alhawamdeh R. Role of gastrointestinal health in managing children with autism spectrum disorder. World Journal of Clinical Pediatrics. 2023;**12**(4):171

[56] Yule S, Wanik J, Holm EM, Bruder MB, Shanley E, Sherman CQ, et al. Nutritional deficiency disease secondary to ARFID symptoms associated with autism and the broad autism phenotype: A qualitative systematic review of case reports and case series. Journal of the Academy of Nutrition and Dietetics. 2021;**121**(3):467-492

[57] Marinov D, Chamova R, Pancheva R. Micronutrient deficiencies in children with autism spectrum disorders compared to typically developing children—A scoping review. Research in Autism Spectrum Disorders. 2024;**114**:102396

[58] Jiang Y, Dang W, Nie H, Kong X, Jiang Z, Guo J. Omega-3 polyunsaturated fatty acids and/or vitamin D in autism spectrum disorders: A systematic review. Frontiers in Psychiatry. 2023;**14**:1238973

[59] Veselinović A, Petrović S, Žikić V, Subotić M, Jakovljević V, Jeremić N, et al. Neuroinflammation in autism and supplementation based on omega-3 polyunsaturated fatty acids: A narrative review. Medicina. 2021;**57**(9):893

[60] Choi S, Hong DK, Choi BY, Suh SW. Zinc in the brain: Friend or foe? International Journal of Molecular Sciences. 2020;**21**(23):8941

[61] Guo M, Zhu J, Yang T, Lai X, Lei Y, Chen J, et al. Vitamin A and vitamin D deficiencies exacerbate symptoms in children with autism spectrum disorders. Nutritional Neuroscience. 2019;**22**(9):637-647

[62] Rostami Haji Abadi M, Neumeyer A, Misra M, Kontulainen S. Bone health in children and youth with ASD: A systematic review and meta-analysis. Osteoporosis International. 2021;**32**(9):1679-1691

[63] Doseděl M, Jirkovský E, Macáková K, Krčmová LK, Javorská L, Pourová J, et al. Vitamin C—Sources, physiological role, kinetics, deficiency, use, toxicity, and determination. Nutrients. 2021;**13**(2):615

[64] Sakamornchai W, Dumrongwongsiri O, Siwarom S. Case report: Vitamin C combined with multiple micronutrient deficiencies is associated with pulmonary arterial hypertension in children with autistic spectrum disorder. Frontiers in Nutrition. 2022;**9**:928026

[65] Robea MA, Luca AC, Ciobica A. Relationship between vitamin deficiencies and co-occurring symptoms in autism spectrum disorder. Medicina. 2020;**56**(5):245

[66] Zhang M, Wu Y, Lu Z, Song M, Huang X, Mi L, et al. Effects of vitamin D supplementation on children with autism spectrum disorder: A systematic review and meta-analysis. Clinical Psychopharmacology and Neuroscience. 2023;**21**(2):240

[67] Jennings L, Basiri R. Amino acids, B vitamins, and choline may independently and collaboratively influence the incidence and core symptoms of autism spectrum disorder. Nutrients. 2022;**14**(14):2896

[68] Barón-Mendoza I, González-Arenas A. Relationship between the effect of polyunsaturated fatty acids (PUFAs) on brain plasticity and the improvement on cognition and behavior in individuals with autism spectrum disorder. Nutritional Neuroscience. 2022;**25**(2):387-410

[69] Parletta N, Niyonsenga T, Duff J. Omega-3 and omega-6 polyunsaturated fatty acid levels and correlations with symptoms in children with attention deficit hyperactivity disorder, autistic spectrum disorder and typically developing controls. PLoS ONE. 2016;**11**(5):e0156432

[70] Lange KW. Omega-3 fatty acids and mental health. Global Health Journal. 2020;**4**(1):18-30

[71] Kaczmarek KA, Dobrzyńska M, Drzymała-Czyż S. Iron, magnesium,

zinc and selenium—The most common elemental deficiencies in children with autism spectrum disorder. Research in Autism Spectrum Disorders. 2024;**110**:102288

[72] Behl S, Mehta S, Pandey MK. Abnormal levels of metal micronutrients and autism spectrum disorder: A perspective review. Frontiers in Molecular Neuroscience. 2020;**13**:586209

[73] Goyal DK, Neil JR, Simmons SD, Mansab F, Benjamin S, Pitfield V. Zinc deficiency in autism: A controlled study. Insights in Biomedicine. 2019;**4**:12

[74] Tsujiguchi H, Miyagi S, Nguyen TT, Hara A, Ono Y, Kambayashi Y, et al. Relationship between autistic traits and nutrient intake among Japanese children and adolescents. Nutrients. 2020;**12**(8):2258

[75] Formosa MM, Christou MA, Mäkitie O. Bone fragility and osteoporosis in children and young adults. Journal of Endocrinological Investigation. 2024;**47**(2):285-298

[76] Guo M, Li L, Zhang Q, Chen L, Dai Y, Liu L, et al. Vitamin and mineral status of children with autism spectrum disorder in Hainan Province of China: Associations with symptoms. Nutritional Neuroscience. 2020;**23**(10):803-810

[77] Fiłon J, Ustymowicz-Farbiszewska J, Krajewska-Kułak E. Analysis of lead, arsenic and calcium content in the hair of children with autism spectrum disorder. BMC Public Health. 2020;**20**:1-8

[78] Mustafa Khalid N, Haron H, Shahar S, Fenech M. Current evidence on the association of micronutrient malnutrition with mild cognitive impairment, frailty, and cognitive frailty among older adults: A scoping review. International Journal of Environmental Research and Public Health. 2022;**19**(23):15722

[79] Moiniafshari K, Gholami M, Dalvand H, Efatpanah M, Rezayi S. Evaluation of functional training along with online nutritional education on autistic children's metabolic status during Covid-19 pandemic—A randomized clinical trial. African Journal of Diabetes Medicine. 1 Feb 2022;**30**(1)

[80] Mottron L, Bzdok D. Autism spectrum heterogeneity: Fact or artifact? Molecular Psychiatry. 2020;**25**(12):3178-3185

[81] Toscano CV, Barros L, Lima AB, Nunes T, Carvalho HM, Gaspar JM. Neuroinflammation in autism spectrum disorders: Exercise as a "pharmacological" tool. Neuroscience and Biobehavioral Reviews. 2021;**129**:63-74

[82] Žigman T, Petković Ramadža D, Šimić G, Barić I. Inborn errors of metabolism associated with autism spectrum disorders: Approaches to intervention. Frontiers in Neuroscience. 2021;**15**:673600

[83] Al-Beltagi M. Autism medical comorbidities. World Journal of Clinical Pediatrics. 2021;**10**(3):15

[84] Cheng N, Rho JM, Masino SA. Metabolic dysfunction underlying autism spectrum disorder and potential treatment approaches. Frontiers in Molecular Neuroscience. 2017;**10**:34

[85] Khaliulin I, Hamoudi W, Amal H. The multifaceted role of mitochondria in autism spectrum disorder. Molecular Psychiatry. Feb 2025;**30**(2):629-650

[86] Rossignol DA, Frye RE. Mitochondrial dysfunction in autism spectrum disorders: A systematic review

and meta-analysis. Molecular Psychiatry. 2012;**17**(3):290-314

[87] Varga NÁ, Pentelényi K, Balicza P, Gézsi A, Reményi V, Hársfalvi V, et al. Mitochondrial dysfunction and autism: Comprehensive genetic analyses of children with autism and mtDNA deletion. Behavioral and Brain Functions. 2018;**14**:1-4

[88] Citrigno L, Muglia M, Qualtieri A, Spadafora P, Cavalcanti F, Pioggia G, et al. The mitochondrial dysfunction hypothesis in autism spectrum disorders: Current status and future perspectives. International Journal of Molecular Sciences. 2020;**21**(16):5785

[89] Frye RE, Rincon N, McCarty PJ, Brister D, Scheck AC, Rossignol DA. Biomarkers of mitochondrial dysfunction in autism spectrum disorder: A systematic review and meta-analysis. Neurobiology of Disease. 2024;**197**:106520

[90] Chen L, Shi XJ, Liu H, Mao X, Gui LN, Wang H, et al. Oxidative stress marker aberrations in children with autism spectrum disorder: A systematic review and meta-analysis of 87 studies (N= 9109). Translational Psychiatry. 2021;**11**(1):15

[91] Thorsen M, Bilenberg N, Thorsen L, Michel TM. Oxidative stress in adults with autism spectrum disorder: A case control study. Journal of Autism and Developmental Disorders. 2022;**52**:275-282

[92] Bjørklund G, Meguid NA, El-Bana MA, Tinkov AA, Saad K, Dadar M, et al. Oxidative stress in autism spectrum disorder. Molecular Neurobiology. 2020;**57**:2314-2332

[93] Liu X, Lin J, Zhang H, Khan NU, Zhang J, Tang X, et al. Oxidative stress in autism spectrum disorder—Current progress of mechanisms and biomarkers. Frontiers in Psychiatry. 2022;**13**:813304

[94] Frye RE, Delatorre R, Taylor H, Slattery J, Melnyk S, Chowdhury N, et al. Redox metabolism abnormalities in autistic children associated with mitochondrial disease. Translational Psychiatry. 2013;**3**(6):e273

[95] Bjørklund G, Tinkov AA, Hosnedlová B, Kizek R, Ajsuvakova OP, Chirumbolo S, et al. The role of glutathione redox imbalance in autism spectrum disorder: A review. Free Radical Biology and Medicine. 2020;**160**:149-162

[96] Bakulski KM, Dou JF, Feinberg JI, Aung MT, Ladd-Acosta C, Volk HE, et al. Autism-associated DNA methylation at birth from multiple tissues is enriched for autism genes in the early autism risk longitudinal investigation. Frontiers in Molecular Neuroscience. 2021;**14**:775390

[97] Stathopoulos S, Gaujoux R, Lindeque Z, Mahony C, Van Der Colff R, Van Der Westhuizen F, et al. DNA methylation associated with mitochondrial dysfunction in a South African autism spectrum disorder cohort. Autism Research. 2020;**13**(7):1079-1093

[98] Roufael M, Bitar T, Sacre Y, Andres C, Hleihel W. Folate–Methionine Cycle Disruptions in ASD Patients and Possible Interventions: A Systematic Review. Genes. 2023;**14**(3):709

[99] James SJ, Cutler P, Melnyk S, Jernigan S, Janak L, Gaylor DW, et al. Metabolic biomarkers of increased oxidative stress and impaired methylation capacity in children with autism. The American Journal of Clinical Nutrition. 2004;**80**(6):1611-1617

[100] Neggers Y. The relationship between folic acid and risk of autism spectrum disorders. Healthcare. 2014;**2**(4):429-444

[101] Main PA, Angley MT, Thomas P, O'Doherty CE, Fenech M. Folate and methionine metabolism in autism: A systematic review. The American Journal of Clinical Nutrition. 2010;**91**(6):1598-1620

[102] Belardo A, Gevi F, Zolla L. The concomitant lower concentrations of vitamins B6, B9 and B12 may cause methylation deficiency in autistic children. Journal of Nutritional Biochemistry. 2019;**70**:38-46

[103] Lintas C. Linking genetics to epigenetics: The role of folate and folate-related pathways in neurodevelopmental disorders. Clinical Genetics. 2019;**95**(2):241-252

[104] Maltsev D, Kurchenko A, Marushko Y, Yuriev S. Biochemical profile of children with autism spectrum disorders associated with genetic deficiency of the folate cycle. Biochimica Clinica. 2023;**47**(2):133

[105] Skalny AV, Skalny AA, Lobanova YN, Korobeinikova TV, Ajsuvakova OP, Notova SV, et al. Serum amino acid spectrum in children with autism spectrum disorder (ASD). Research in Autism Spectrum Disorders. 2020;**77**:101605

[106] Smith AM, King JJ, West PR, Ludwig MA, Donley EL, Burrier RE, et al. Amino acid dysregulation metabotypes: Potential biomarkers for diagnosis and individualized treatment for subtypes of autism spectrum disorder. Biological Psychiatry. 2019;**85**(4):345-354

[107] Brister D, Rose S, Delhey L, Tippett M, Jin Y, Gu H, et al. Metabolomic signatures of autism spectrum disorder. Journal of Personalized Medicine. 2022;**12**(10):1727

[108] Ferraro S, Saielli L, Biganzoli D, Tosi M, Guidi L, Longo R, et al. Amino acid patterns in children with autistic spectrum disorder: A preliminary biochemical evaluation. Nutrients. 2025;**17**(2):274

[109] Chen WX, Chen YR, Peng MZ, Liu X, Cai YN, Huang ZF, et al. Plasma amino acid profile in children with autism spectrum disorder in Southern China: Analysis of 110 cases. Journal of Autism and Developmental Disorders. 2024;**54**(4):1567-1581

[110] Zou M, Li D, Wang L, Li L, Xie S, Liu Y, et al. Identification of amino acid dysregulation as a potential biomarker for autism spectrum disorder in China. Neurotoxicity Research. 2020;**38**:992-1000

[111] Hollestein V, Poelmans G, Forde NJ, Beckmann CF, Ecker C, Mann C, et al. Excitatory/inhibitory imbalance in autism: The role of glutamate and GABA gene-sets in symptoms and cortical brain structure. Translational Psychiatry. 2023;**13**(1):18

[112] Al-Otaish H, Al-Ayadhi L, Bjørklund G, Chirumbolo S, Urbina MA, El-Ansary A. Relationship between absolute and relative ratios of glutamate, glutamine and GABA and severity of autism spectrum disorder. Metabolic Brain Disease. 2018;**33**:843-854

[113] Nisar S, Bhat AA, Masoodi T, Hashem S, Akhtar S, Ali TA, et al. Genetics of glutamate and its receptors in autism spectrum disorder. Molecular Psychiatry. 2022;**27**(5):2380-2392

[114] Blum K, Bowirrat A, Sunder K, Thanos PK, Hanna C, Gold MS, et al. Dopamine dysregulation in reward and autism spectrum disorder. Brain Sciences. 2024;**14**(7):733

[115] Kuo HY, Liu FC. Pathophysiological studies of monoaminergic neurotransmission systems in valproic acid-induced model of autism spectrum disorder. Biomedicine. 2022;**10**(3):560

[116] Wegiel J, Chadman K, London E, Wisniewski T, Wegiel J. Contribution of the serotonergic system to developmental brain abnormalities in autism spectrum disorder. Autism Research. Jul 2024;**17**(7):1300-1321

[117] Kosillo P, Bateup HS. Dopaminergic dysregulation in syndromic autism spectrum disorders: Insights from genetic mouse models. Frontiers in Neural Circuits. 2021;**15**:700968

[118] Kurokawa S, Nomura K, Miyaho K, Sanada K, Iwamoto C, Naraoka M, et al. Gastrointestinal symptoms and sensory abnormalities associated with behavioral problems in children with neurodevelopmental disorders. Autism Research. 2021;**14**(9):1996-2001

[119] Holingue C, Poku O, Pfeiffer D, Murray S, Fallin MD. Gastrointestinal concerns in children with autism spectrum disorder: A qualitative study of family experiences. Autism. 2022;**26**(7):1698-1711

[120] Holingue C, Pfeiffer D, Ludwig NN, Reetzke R, Hong JS, Kalb LG, et al. Prevalence of gastrointestinal symptoms among autistic individuals, with and without co-occurring intellectual disability. Autism Research. 2023;**16**(8):1609-1618

[121] Morais LH, Schreiber HL IV, Mazmanian SK. The gut microbiota–brain axis in behaviour and brain disorders. Nature Reviews Microbiology. 2021;**19**(4):241-255

[122] Yang J, Fu X, Liao X, Li Y. Effects of gut microbial-based treatments on gut microbiota, behavioral symptoms, and gastrointestinal symptoms in children with autism spectrum disorder: A systematic review. Psychiatry Research. 2020;**293**:113471

[123] Ding X, Xu Y, Zhang X, Zhang L, Duan G, Song C, et al. Gut microbiota changes in patients with autism spectrum disorders. Journal of Psychiatric Research. 2020;**129**:149-159

[124] Wu T, Wang H, Lu W, Zhai Q, Zhang Q, Yuan W, et al. Potential of gut microbiome for detection of autism spectrum disorder. Microbial Pathogenesis. 2020;**149**:104568

[125] Liu F, Li J, Wu F, Zheng H, Peng Q, Zhou H. Altered composition and function of intestinal microbiota in autism spectrum disorders: A systematic review. Translational Psychiatry. 2019;**9**(1):43

[126] Bezawada N, Phang TH, Hold GL, Hansen R. Autism spectrum disorder and the gut microbiota in children: A systematic review. Annals of Nutrition and Metabolism. 2020;**76**(1):16-29

[127] Iannone LF, Preda A, Blottière HM, Clarke G, Albani D, Belcastro V, et al. Microbiota-gut brain axis involvement in neuropsychiatric disorders. Expert Review of Neurotherapeutics. 2019;**19**(10):1037-1050

[128] Yang W, Cong Y. Gut microbiota-derived metabolites in the regulation of host immune responses and immune-related inflammatory diseases. Cellular and Molecular Immunology. 2021;**18**(4):866-877

[129] Wang J, Zhu N, Su X, Gao Y, Yang R. Gut-microbiota-derived metabolites maintain gut and systemic immune homeostasis. Cells. 2023;**12**(5):793

[130] Ahmed H, Leyrolle Q, Koistinen V, Kärkkäinen O, Layé S, Delzenne N, et al. Microbiota-derived metabolites as drivers of gut–brain communication. Gut Microbes. 2022;**14**(1):2102878

[131] Liu S, Li E, Sun Z, Fu D, Duan G, Jiang M, et al. Altered gut microbiota and short chain fatty acids in Chinese children with autism spectrum disorder. Scientific Reports. 2019;**9**(1):287

[132] Cao X, Liu K, Liu J, Liu YW, Xu L, Wang H, et al. Dysbiotic gut microbiota and dysregulation of cytokine profile in children and teens with autism spectrum disorder. Frontiers in Neuroscience. 2021;**15**:635925

[133] Lagod PP, Abdelli LS, Naser SA. An in vivo model of propionic acid-rich diet-induced gliosis and neuro-inflammation in mice (FVB/N-Tg (GFAPGFP) 14Mes/J): A potential link to autism spectrum disorder. International Journal of Molecular Sciences. 2024;**25**(15):8093

[134] Fanelli G, Franke B, De Witte W, et al. Insulinopathies of the brain? Genetic overlap between somatic insulin-related and neuropsychiatric disorders. Translational Psychiatry. 2022;**12**:59

[135] Hoirisch-Clapauch S, Nardi AE. Autism spectrum disorders: Let's talk about glucose? Translational Psychiatry. 2019;**9**(1):51

[136] Manco M, Guerrera S, Ravà L, Ciofi degli Atti M, Di Vara S, Valeri G, et al. Cross-sectional investigation of insulin resistance in youths with autism spectrum disorder. Any role for reduced brain glucose metabolism? Translational Psychiatry. 2021;**11**(1):229

[137] Cortese S, Gabellone A, Marzulli L, Iturmendi-Sabater I, de La Chica-Duarte D, Pique IM, et al. Association between autism spectrum disorder and diabetes: Systematic review and meta-analysis. Neuroscience and Biobehavioral Reviews. 2022;**136**:104592

[138] Hodges H, Fealko C, Soares N. Autism spectrum disorder: Definition, epidemiology, causes, and clinical evaluation. Translational Pediatrics. 2020;**9**(Suppl. 1):S55

[139] De Vivo DC, Trifiletti RR, Jacobson RI, Ronen GM, Behmand RA, Harik SI. Defective glucose transport across the blood-brain barrier as a cause of persistent hypoglycorrhachia, seizures, and developmental delay. The New England Journal of Medicine. 1991;**325**(10):703-709

[140] Al-Bishri WM. Glucose transporter 1 deficiency, AMP-activated protein kinase activation and immune dysregulation in autism spectrum disorder: Novel biomarker sources for clinical diagnosis. Saudi Journal of Biological Sciences. 2023;**30**(12):103849

[141] Wu X, Wang C, Wang J, Zhu M, Yao Y, Liu J. Hypoxia preconditioning protects neuronal cells against traumatic brain injury through stimulation of glucose transport mediated by HIF-1α/GLUTs signaling pathway in rat. Neurosurgical Review. 2021;**44**(1):411-422

[142] Wang L, Pavlou S, Du X, Bhuckory M, Xu H, Chen M. Glucose transporter 1 critically controls microglial activation through facilitating glycolysis. Molecular Neurodegeneration. 2019;**14**:1-5

[143] Meyer N, Richter N, Fan Z, Siemonsmeier G, Pivneva T, Jordan P, et al. Oligodendrocytes in the mouse corpus callosum maintain axonal function by delivery of glucose. Cell Reports. 2018;**22**(9):2383-2394

[144] Winkler EA, Nishida Y, Sagare AP, Rege SV, Bell RD, Perlmutter D, et al. GLUT1 reductions exacerbate Alzheimer's disease vasculo-neuronal dysfunction and degeneration. Nature Neuroscience. 2015;**18**(4):521-530

[145] Mitelman SA, Bralet MC, Mehmet Haznedar M, Hollander E, Shihabuddin L, Hazlett EA, et al. Positron emission tomography assessment of cerebral glucose metabolic rates in autism spectrum disorder and schizophrenia. Brain Imaging and Behavior. 2018;**12**:532-546

[146] Courchesne E, Gazestani VH, Lewis NE. Prenatal origins of ASD: The when, what, and how of ASD development. Trends in Neurosciences. 2020;**43**(5):326-342

[147] Puljko B, Štracak M, Kalanj-Bognar S, Todorić Laidlaw I, Mlinac-Jerkovic K. Gangliosides and cholesterol: Dual regulators of neuronal membrane framework in autism spectrum disorder. International Journal of Molecular Sciences. 2025;**26**(3):1322

[148] Esposito CM, Buoli M, Ciappolino V, Agostoni C, Brambilla P. The role of cholesterol and fatty acids in the etiology and diagnosis of autism spectrum disorders. International Journal of Molecular Sciences. 2021;**22**(7):3550

[149] Martín MG, Pfrieger F, Dotti CG. Cholesterol in brain disease: Sometimes determinant and frequently implicated. EMBO Reports. 2014;**15**(10):1036-1052

[150] Qasem H, Al-Ayadhi L, Bjørklund G, Chirumbolo S, El-Ansary A. Impaired lipid metabolism markers to assess the risk of neuroinflammation in autism spectrum disorder. Metabolic Brain Disease. 2018;**33**:1141-1153

[151] Yui K, Imataka G, Yoshihara S. Lipid-based molecules on signaling pathways in autism spectrum disorder. International Journal of Molecular Sciences. 2022;**23**(17):9803

[152] Wong C, Crawford DA. Lipid signalling in the pathology of autism spectrum disorders. In: Comprehensive Guide to Autism. Vol. 18. New York, NY: Springer; 2014. pp. 1259-1283

[153] Kang DW, Adams JB, Gregory AC, Borody T, Chittick L, Fasano A, et al. Microbiota transfer therapy alters gut ecosystem and improves gastrointestinal and autism symptoms: An open-label study. Microbiome. 2017;**5**:1-6

[154] Karhu E, Zukerman R, Eshraghi RS, Mittal J, Deth RC, Castejon AM, et al. Nutritional interventions for autism spectrum disorder. Nutrition Reviews. 2020;**78**(7):515-531

[155] Adams JB, Bhargava A, Coleman DM, Frye RE, Rossignol DA. Ratings of the effectiveness of nutraceuticals for autism spectrum disorders: Results of a national survey. Journal of Personalized Medicine. 2021;**11**(9):878

Chapter 2

# Perspective Chapter: Leveraging Machine Learning for Early Detection of Autism Spectrum Disorder through Motion Analysis

*Roberta Simeoli and Davide Marocco*

## Abstract

Autism spectrum disorder (ASD) is traditionally diagnosed through extended behavioral observations. New evidence suggests that motor abnormalities may underline the disorder and serve as computational markers, potentially improving both assessment and diagnostic processes. In this context, machine learning (ML)-based approaches are paving the way for faster, more objective methods of early ASD detection by analyzing these transparent, measurable indicators. This chapter provides an overview of theories supporting these new assessment perspectives and recent ML applications that can assist ASD diagnostic processes through the analysis of motor data collected *via* digital devices, such as tablets with touchscreen sensors or wearable sensors. Offering a comprehensive and critical view of these innovations, this chapter highlights the potential contributions of ML-based motor analysis in detecting autism biomarkers, the implications for early diagnosis, and the ongoing challenges in integrating these tools into clinical practice.

**Keywords:** autism spectrum disorder, machine learning, motion analysis, early diagnosis, motor patterns, artificial neural networks

## 1. Introduction

Autism was first described in 1943 by Leo Kanner [1], who identified some fundamental characteristics of the disorder, including social isolation, repetitive behaviors, and difficulties in motor regulation and anticipation. Over the years, subsequent studies have expanded our understanding of autism, revealing that these deficits may be linked not only to social and communicative impairments but also to problems in integrating sensory and proprioceptive information. This observation has paved the way for interpreting autism within the theoretical framework of predictive coding.

Predictive coding, as proposed by Karl Friston et al. [2], posits that the brain operates as a hierarchical Bayesian inference system, continuously generating and updating predictions about sensory inputs. In this model, perception and action emerge from the dynamic interplay between top-down expectations and bottom-up sensory evidence. When discrepancies arise between predictions and actual sensory inputs, the brain revises its internal models to minimize prediction error. In autism, however, this predictive capacity appears to be altered due to an "aberrant precision" of sensory information. This imbalance—where excessive reliance on sensory inputs overshadows internal expectations—leads to difficulties in integrating bottom-up inputs with top-down models, resulting in hypersensitivity to stimuli and challenges in adapting to environmental changes. Such dysfunctions affect multiple cognitive, perceptual, and notably, motor processes.

One particularly significant consequence of this altered predictive mechanism is its impact on motor control. Research by Lawson et al. [3, 4] indicates that individuals with autism spectrum disorder (ASD) struggle to filter and select relevant stimuli, undermining their ability to plan and coordinate movements smoothly. This impairment manifests as atypical motor behaviors, including difficulties in movement synchronization, postural alterations, and deficits in motor anticipation. Neuroimaging studies have further substantiated these findings by revealing reduced cortical connectivity [5, 6], which may reflect underlying anomalies in inter-regional brain communication.

Autism spectrum disorder is now recognized as a neurodevelopmental condition characterized by deficits in social communication and interaction, alongside restricted and repetitive behaviors—ranging from stereotyped motor movements and insistence on sameness to an unusual response to sensory stimuli. Importantly, motor impairments in ASD have been observed from very early in development [7, 8], become more pronounced over time [9], and significantly impact the quality of life and social development [10]. Abnormalities have been documented in various motor domains, including walking patterns [11–13], hand movements such as reaching and grasping [14, 15], and eye-hand coordination [16].

The growing body of evidence underscores the need for more reliable and earlier diagnostic processes for ASD. Early detection is critical—not only for accurate diagnosis but also for timely intervention, which is vital for improving outcomes for both children and their families [17]. Traditionally, ASD diagnosis relies on time-consuming clinical assessments, such as the Autism Diagnostic Observation Schedule [18], with reliable identification often occurring after the age of three. The inherent variability of symptoms further complicates the diagnostic process.

Against this backdrop, recent technological advances have opened new avenues for objective assessment. Computer-assisted analysis, particularly through machine learning (ML) techniques, has shown promise in identifying specific behavioral markers, such as distinctive motor patterns and eye-gaze dynamics, that may serve as early indicators of ASD. Methods ranging from artificial neural networks (ANN) and support vector machines (SVM) to decision trees have been applied to autism-related datasets, with the aim of maximizing the discriminative power between affected and typically developing individuals. Studies using wearable sensors and video analysis systems integrated with AI (e.g., [19, 20]) further demonstrate the potential of these approaches to quantify motor abnormalities and unravel the neurobiological underpinnings of ASD.

In summary, integrating the insights from predictive coding and the observed motor impairments in autism not only enriches our theoretical understanding of the disorder but also highlights the critical role of innovative, ML-based methodologies in early detection. By automating the analysis of movement data, the proposed approach aims to improve early diagnosis and foster a more comprehensive understanding of the neurophysiological mechanisms underlying autism, ultimately contributing to more effective and timely interventions.

## 2. Machine learning clinical application

The application of ML to clinical datasets is increasingly recognized as a powerful resource for enhancing diagnostic procedures, particularly in the context of autism spectrum disorder (ASD). Before delving into the specifics of ML in ASD diagnosis, it is important to briefly explain how ML functions and how these systems can support the diagnostic process.

ML enables the development of algorithms that learn from data by identifying complex patterns or features, which can then be used to classify new observations. In supervised learning, for example, a model is trained on a dataset where each subject is labeled (e.g., as having ASD or being typically developing [TD]). The algorithm learns the distinctive features that differentiate these groups and uses these learned rules to predict the diagnostic class of new subjects [21]. In contrast, unsupervised learning does not rely on labeled data; rather, it seeks to uncover hidden structures or natural groupings within the data. Techniques such as principal component analysis (PCA), k-means clustering, and other dimensionality reduction methods are employed to discover new patterns, which can be especially valuable in a heterogeneous disorder like ASD.

From a clinical perspective, the ML-based diagnostic procedure generally involves a training phase—where a classifier is developed using a well-defined dataset—and a testing phase, during which the model's predictive performance is evaluated on new data. For instance, a study might utilize movement data collected *via* wearable sensors to train an algorithm to recognize the motor abnormalities characteristic of ASD. Once trained, the model can then be applied to new cases to determine whether the observed pattern corresponds to ASD or TD, thus supporting early diagnosis [17]. Moreover, the use of pattern recognition methods in ML extends beyond merely assigning a diagnostic label; it also holds the potential to identify novel, objective measures that could contribute to a refined phenotypic definition of the disorder. Techniques such as support vector machines (SVM) or artificial neural networks (ANN) have been used to pinpoint specific irregularities in body movements or eye-gaze behavior, offering deeper insights into the variability of ASD.

The reliability and effectiveness of predictive models depend heavily on both the quality and quantity of the training data and on the ability to select the most relevant features. High-dimensional datasets often contain irrelevant, noisy, or redundant information, which can hinder model performance and increase computational cost. Therefore, feature selection techniques are employed to reduce dimensionality, thereby enhancing classification accuracy and efficiency [22]. To evaluate the performance of ML models, standard metrics such as accuracy (the percentage of correctly classified cases), sensitivity (the ability to correctly identify true positives), and specificity (the ability to correctly identify true negatives) are used. A common challenge in ML is overfitting—where a model becomes too tailored to the training data and fails to generalize to new cases. To mitigate overfitting, cross-validation techniques such as k-fold, leave-one-out (LOO), and leave-one-subject-out (LOSO) are employed, offering robust estimates of a model's generalization performance.

In summary, it appears that automated analysis and pattern recognition can significantly support the ASD diagnostic process. These methods not only can facilitate early and accurate diagnosis but also can provide the potential to uncover new objective markers, contributing to a more comprehensive understanding and phenotypic redefinition of autism.

Based on these findings, the following paragraphs will illustrate how, in recent years, technology and ML analysis have proven to be valuable in the clinical field of autism assessment by using transparent data on eye movement and overall body movement.

### 2.1 Body motion-related features extraction

ASD symptomatology is believed to stem, in part, from impairments in early learning processes that affect active perception, planning, and coordination [23]. Inefficient processing of external information can lead to delays in cognitive, language, and social development. By tracking how individuals with ASD move within their environment, researchers can identify specific motor patterns characteristic of the disorder. ML systems have demonstrated the capacity to extract these often "invisible" and objective features, thus supporting early diagnosis. Numerous studies have leveraged various motion tasks to reveal subtle differences between ASD and typically developing (TD) individuals.

A considerable body of work has focused on reach-and-grasp tasks as a means to capture kinematic abnormalities in ASD. For example, Emanuele et al. [24] used an optoelectronic motion capture system with passive markers placed symmetrically on the upper limbs and on the manubrium to record reach-and-grasp movements, achieving an accuracy of up to 95% using a support vector machine (SVM) algorithm. Similarly, Perego et al. [19] recorded kinematic variables during a reach-and-throw task using eight infrared cameras and applied SVM with 10-fold cross-validation, achieving 92.5% accuracy. Cavallo et al. [25] also captured reach-and-grasp movements *via* a camera-based motion capture system with hand markers, and, using an SVM, they reached an accuracy of 75%. Crippa et al. [26] collected 17 kinematic measures with an optoelectronic system and passive markers, then applied an SVM classifier combined with a Fisher discriminant ratio (FDR)-based feature selection approach, which yielded a maximum classification accuracy of 96.7% using seven features related to goal-oriented movement phases. Together, these studies illustrate that despite using different data capture tools and classification models, reach-and-grasp tasks provide reliable markers for differentiating ASD from TD children.

Another promising approach involves imitation tasks, which examine the nuances of finger movement. Vabalas et al. [20, 27] and Li et al. [28] explored finger kinematics during a pointing imitation task by collecting data with motion sensors attached to the distal phalange of the index finger, sometimes in conjunction with remote eye trackers. These studies extracted features such as velocity, acceleration, jerk, and movement amplitude. They reported classification accuracies of approximately 73% for movement data and 70% for eye-gaze data, with an overall improvement to 78% when datasets were combined using SVM with nested cross-validation. In a complementary study, Li et al. [28] extracted 40 features and compared various classifiers (Naive Bayes, SVM, decision trees, and random forests) along with different feature selection methods. Their best result reached an accuracy of 86.7%, highlighting the importance of selecting the most appropriate model and features for each dataset.

Ecological tools that are widely available in everyday life, such as smart tablets, have also been used to extract significant motion features in a naturalistic setting. Anzulewicz et al. [29] used a smart tablet equipped with a touchscreen and inertial sensors to record finger kinematics during gameplay, analyzing 262 data points with various algorithms to achieve a classification accuracy of 93%. Similarly, Simeoli et al. [30] collected finger motion coordinates during a simple cognitive task administered *via* a tablet and extracted 12 motion features (e.g., acceleration, velocity, straightness, and directional changes) using a feedforward multilayer perceptron artificial neural network (ANN), which also reached 93% accuracy.

Additional research has focused on pose estimation, which involves extracting features related to the movement of various body parts. Raya et al. [31, 32] used a camera to estimate real-time body pose by analyzing 25 joints during a virtual multisensory experience. Applying SVM with leave-one-subject-out (LOSO) cross-validation, they achieved an accuracy of about 83% based on head and trunk parameters. Robles et al. [33] extracted 27 features—including hand, head, and gaze behavior—using the HTC VIVE Pro Eye VR system combined with the Tobii XR SDK. They compared logistic regression, SVM, and ANN models through fivefold cross-validation, with the ANN yielding 93.3% accuracy on a randomly grouped dataset (versus 86.7% on matched datasets). Other studies include Kojovic et al. [34], who used OpenPose for 2D pose estimation during ADOS sessions with a convolutional neural network (CNN) achieving 80.9% accuracy; Zhao et al. [35], who employed OpenFace 2.0 to extract head movement time series during conversation with a decision tree classifier reaching 92.11% accuracy; and Li et al. [36], who used a force plate to extract center-of-pressure features and found that naïve Bayes achieved 90% accuracy, outperforming other classifiers.

Current research indicates that reach-and-grasp tasks, imitation exercises, and ecological tools like tablets can serve as effective markers for differentiating children with ASD from those with typical development. Motion capture techniques combined with ML algorithms, especially SVM and ANN, have demonstrated high classification accuracy. Moreover, posture and body movement analysis using cameras and sensors has yielded promising results, highlighting the potential benefits of integrating multiple approaches to improve diagnostic accuracy.

### 2.2 Eye motion-related feature extraction

Eye tracking has received significant attention in ASD research due to the hallmark ocular gaze abnormalities observed in the disorder [37]. This technology objectively measures fixations, saccades, and blinks, allowing for detailed scanpath analysis that represents gaze behavior as a sequence of fixations and saccades. Several studies have focused on visual fixation times on specific areas-of-interest (AOI) during various tasks. For instance, Zhao et al. [35] used a head-mounted eye tracker during face-to-face conversations and applied multiple classification methods (SVM, LDA, decision trees, and random forests) to features combining fixation time and session length, achieving up to 92.31% accuracy. Liu et al. [38] examined face-scanning patterns during a face recognition task using SVM, reaching 88.51% accuracy, and identified key facial areas that accounted for most of the discriminative power between TD and ASD groups. Jiang et al. [39] combined task, face, and gaze features using a random forest classifier, which raised sensitivity to 91.3%, while Wan et al. [40] reported 85.1% accuracy using SVM on fixation data collected during video observation. Broader approaches have also been explored: Liaqat et al. [41] used a multilayer perceptron (MLP) on free-viewing eye fixation coordinates, achieving 67.23% accuracy; Alcañiz et al. [42] extracted four eye-tracking variables during a virtual experience and, using SVM, reached 86% accuracy; Elbattah et al. [43] employed an autoencoder for feature extraction and k-means clustering to confirm that scan-paths could be grouped coherently; and Tsuchiya et al. [44] demonstrated that combining AOI rate and count scores *via* a best-fit algorithm could discriminate between ASD and TD individuals with

78% accuracy. Additional work by Cilia et al. [45] applied a CNN to analyze point-of-gaze data, achieving 71% accuracy, while Kanhirakadavath and Chandran [46] focused on dynamic eye movement features such as velocity, acceleration, and jerk using a deep neural network (DNN), which improved accuracy to 78.6% after data augmentation. Finally, Lin et al. [47] proposed a novel technique combining eye movement data with ML algorithms in a virtual reality setting to predict high levels of autistic traits, with random forest, decision tree, and gradient boosting decision tree models achieving up to 70% accuracy—random forest performing best in follow-up experiments.

Eye tracking has proven to be a valuable tool in ASD research, offering objective measurements of gaze behavior that can aid in distinguishing ASD from typical development. Studies leveraging fixation patterns, saccadic movements, and AOI-based analyses have achieved high classification accuracy, particularly when combined with machine learning models such as SVM, random forests, and deep neural networks. Moreover, integrating eye-tracking data with additional features, including task-specific and dynamic eye movement metrics, has further enhanced classification performance. These findings suggest that eye tracking, especially when combined with advanced computational techniques, holds significant potential for improving ASD detection and assessment.

By synthesizing these various approaches—from kinematic analyses in reach-and-grasp tasks to ecological measurements *via* smart tablets and detailed eye-tracking studies—it becomes evident the multifaceted potential of ML in uncovering objective biomarkers for ASD. Summarized in **Tables 1** and **2**, these methods have demonstrated valuable accuracy in classifying ASD and TD. Together, these methodologies contribute not only to early and accurate diagnosis but also to a refined understanding of the disorder's heterogeneous phenotype.

| **Eye motion data** | **SVM** | | **ANN** | | **OTHERS** | |
|---|---|---|---|---|---|---|
| **Features** | **AOI** | **Scanpath** | **AOI** | **Scanpath** | **AOI** | **Scanpath** |
| Num. of studies | 3 | 1 | 0 | 3 | 1 | 3 |
| Accuracy range | 85–92% | 88% | — | 67–90% | 78 | 70–74% |

*N.B. For articles that reported results from various ML models, we have considered for this table only the model that achieved the highest accuracy level.*

**Table 1.**
*Eye motion data results. The table presents the overall results of the studies related to eye motion analysis. Results are arranged based on the ML method used (SVM; ANN; others) and the type of features analyzed (AOI; scanpath).*

| **Body motion data** | **SVM** | | **ANN** | | **OTHERS** | |
|---|---|---|---|---|---|---|
| **Tools** | **Camera** | **Sensor** | **Camera** | **Sensor** | **Camera** | **Sensor** |
| Num. of studies | 5 | 2 | 2 | 1 | 0 | 4 |
| Accuracy range | 75–100% | 70–73% | 80–93% | 93% | — | 67–93% |

*N.B. For articles that report results from various ML models, we have considered for this table only the model that achieved the highest accuracy level.*

**Table 2.**
*Body motion data results. The table presents the overall results of the studies related to body motion analysis. Results are arranged based on the ML method used (SVM; ANN; others) and the type of recording tool method (camera; motion sensor).*

## 3. Discussion

In recent decades the clinical approach to assessing and diagnosing ASD has been based on measuring several explicit behavioral variables, assuming a qualitative value. Although ASD diagnosis and assessment have traditionally relied on standardized tools based on direct behavioral observation in structured settings—such as the Autism Diagnostic Observation Schedule (ADOS [18])—it is now evident that these tools primarily focus on analyzing communication and social interaction, leaving other aspects unexplored, such as sensory difficulties, motor alterations, and interaction with the environment.

For this reason, researchers have been trying to identify quantitative measures of the disorder in the last few years.

In this scenario, embodied cognition theory and predictive coding principle [2, 48] served as a theoretical framework for a new methodological approach focusing on sensory processing analysis and motor abnormalities and general body-world interaction as potential symptomatology indicators.

Many recent studies have raised the problem of categorizing and recognizing autism through these measures, suggesting the exploitation of the potential of the latest technological advances and artificial learning methods [49].

Some of these studies fully fit into this framework, trying to delve into the topic and specifically aiming at identifying quantitative measures of the disorder and their respective threshold values [21].

The studies discussed here highlight that the use of non-invasive technologies, integrated with advanced analytical models, could enhance ASD assessment by making it more objective and ecologically valid. Although the methodologies used are highly heterogeneous in terms of setting, types of data collected, and analytical techniques, a common trend emerges: interactive devices, such as serious games and tablets, allow for the collection of diagnostic information, even in very young children or those with communication difficulties [29, 30].

This perspective not only has the potential to improve early diagnosis but also offers new insights into the pathophysiology of ASD. For example, spatial movement analysis has revealed distinctive features that may be correlated with symptom severity. Some studies have identified differences in eye movements between individuals with ASD and typically developing subjects, although findings remain inconsistent due to varying methodologies [50]. Other studies have demonstrated that parameters such as fixation duration and saccade frequency can be used to distinguish children with ASD based on the type of visual stimulus presented [51]. Furthermore, when analyses are restricted to specific facial areas, classification accuracy improves significantly [35, 38–40].

From a more purely clinical perspective, we can highlight how some of these studies have attempted to describe these ASD-specific movement patterns to gain insights into their functioning and, even more, to explore possible etiopathogenetic explanations. For example, Simeoli et al. [30] observed these features in detail to understand how they appear between groups. Their results revealed that autism motor patterns are characterized by low linearity of movements. The authors illustrated how the ASD group reached a low level of STH and a high level of DC, meaning their trajectories were not straight and were marked by many changes of direction. Furthermore, the average length of their trajectories was lower than that of the TD group, indicating more fragmented movements.

The description of these movements suggests that individuals with autism make greater moment-by-moment adjustments to their progressive movements compared to the neurotypical group [52–54]. Similarly, Whyatt and Craig [54] demonstrated that ASD children made multiple corrective movements during their motion, reaching greater velocity at the end of their movement.

These results support the idea of a fundamental deficit in the prospective control of movement [55–57]. This deficit would manifest through the interruption of anticipatory (feedforward) mechanisms [58, 59] or feedback reafferences [53] during goal-directed actions. Deficits in perceiving others' intentions and in fluid selective attention to appropriate stimuli for programming consistent movement within the external environment are well-documented in autism [60, 61].

All these findings support the idea of a deficit in sensorimotor timing integration that affects the perception–action process and the ability to understand the social environment. If the proprioceptive feedback that allows for online movement guidance is interrupted, movement control errors can occur, resulting in an abnormal motor signature that we propose as a potential marker for children with ASD.

All of this suggests that these types of measurements are not only useful for recognizing the disorder but also for gaining a deeper understanding of it.

Although these findings are promising, several critical issues remain to be addressed to ensure their clinical applicability. One of the main limitations highlighted in the literature is the small sample size in many studies, which may compromise the reliability and generalizability of the results [25–27]. Studies conducted on small samples risk generating weak results, particularly in terms of representing the general population. Some researchers have attempted to mitigate this issue through data augmentation techniques or cross-validation strategies, such as leave-one-out (LOO), which improves classification accuracy without reducing the available data. However, this challenge remains an open question.

Another critical aspect concerns sample selection. Many studies have used highly homogeneous groups, excluding individuals with motor or cognitive comorbidities. While this approach reduces the risk of confounding factors, it may limit the applicability of results to the real clinical population, which is highly heterogeneous. To improve the generalizability of models, it would be beneficial to include participants with varying severity levels and from different cultural and biological backgrounds. Additionally, comparing ASD with other neurodevelopmental disorders, such as attention-deficit/hyperactivity disorder (ADHD), could help identify more specific biomarkers for ASD [2, 53].

Therefore, future research should aim to integrate multiple data sources to improve diagnostic accuracy. Combining eye movement analysis with physiological and behavioral measures—such as brain activity, skin conductance, speech analysis, and body movements—could provide a more comprehensive assessment of ASD risk. This multimodal approach could represent a significant step forward in improving diagnoses and personalizing interventions.

## 4. Conclusion

In conclusion, the integration of predictive coding theory and embodied cognition into autism research has significantly advanced our understanding of the disorder, particularly in relation to sensory processing and motor control. By conceptualizing autism as a condition involving altered predictive mechanisms, researchers have provided a unifying framework that explains a wide range of behavioral and motor impairments. The notion of "aberrant precision" in sensory processing sheds light on the challenges individuals with ASD face in integrating bottom-up sensory inputs with top-down expectations, leading to atypical responses to environmental stimuli and difficulties in motor planning and execution.

The application of ML techniques to autism research has further reinforced the potential of objective, quantitative measures in improving early diagnosis and assessment. Studies leveraging motion capture, eye tracking, and wearable sensor technology have demonstrated that ASD-specific motor patterns can be identified with high accuracy using advanced computational models such as support vector machines and artificial neural networks. These findings highlight the feasibility of developing automated diagnostic tools that are both efficient and ecologically valid, addressing some of the limitations of traditional behavioral assessments.

Moreover, the identification of distinct motor signatures in ASD has profound implications beyond diagnosis. Understanding how movement abnormalities relate to the broader symptomatology of autism may offer new insights into the neurodevelopmental origins of the disorder and inform tailored interventions. Research on reach-and-grasp tasks, imitation exercises, and spatial movement analysis suggests that motor impairments in ASD may stem from deficits in prospective control, disrupted feedforward mechanisms, and impaired sensorimotor integration. These findings align with broader theories of autism that emphasize atypical information processing, reinforcing the need for interdisciplinary approaches to studying the condition.

Despite these promising advancements, several challenges remain. Many studies suffer from small sample sizes, limiting the generalizability of findings and necessitating replication with larger and more diverse populations. Additionally, the heterogeneity of methodologies used across studies underscores the need for standardization in data collection and analysis protocols. Future research should focus on refining classification models, improving feature selection techniques, and integrating multimodal data sources to enhance the reliability and robustness of ASD assessment tools.

Ultimately, by bridging computational neuroscience, cognitive science, and clinical practice, these approaches have the potential to transform how autism is diagnosed and understood. The continued exploration of movement-based biomarkers, in conjunction with predictive coding models, offers a promising avenue for not only improving early detection but also deepening our comprehension of the fundamental mechanisms underlying ASD. As research progresses, the development of accessible, technology-driven diagnostic tools could pave the way for more personalized and effective interventions, ultimately improving the quality of life for individuals with autism and their families.

## Acknowledgements

The author acknowledges the usage of ChatGPT for language polishing of the manuscript. We acknowledge the Project INTENSE (INtegrated Technologies and ENhanced SEnsing for cognition and rehabilitation) and the PRIN Project E-MOVE: Continuous embodied monitoring system for healthy ageing assessment and support Prot. P20225SJNX.

## Conflict of interest

The authors declare no conflict of interest.

## Author details

Roberta Simeoli* and Davide Marocco
Department of Humanistic Studies, Federico II University of Naplese, Italy

*Address all correspondence to: roberta.simeoli@unina.it

## References

[1] Kanner L. Autistic disturbance of affective contact. The Nervous Child. 1943;**2**:217-250

[2] Friston K, Kiebel S. Predictive coding under the free-energy principle. Philosophical Transactions of the Royal Society B: Biological Sciences. 2009;**364**(1521):1211-1221. DOI: 10.1098/rstb.2008.0300

[3] Friston KJ, Lawson R, Frith CD. On hyperpriors and hypopriors: Comment on Pellicano and Burr. Trends in Cognitive Sciences. 2013;**17**:1. DOI: 10.1016/j.tics.2012.11.003

[4] Lawson RP, Rees G, Friston KJ. An aberrant precision account of autism. Frontiers in Human Neuroscience. 2014;**8**:302. DOI: 10.3389/fnhum.2014.00302

[5] Belmonte MK, Allen G, Beckel-Mitchener A, Boulanger LM, Carper RA, Webb SJ. Autism and abnormal development of brain connectivity. The Journal of Neuroscience: The Official Journal of the Society for Neuroscience. 2004;**24**(42):9228-9231. DOI: 10.1523/JNEUROSCI.3340-04.2004

[6] Just MA, Keller TA, Malave VL, Kana RK, Varma S. Autism as a neural systems disorder: A theory of frontal-posterior underconnectivity. Neuroscience and Biobehavioral Reviews. 2012;**36**(4):1292-1313. DOI: 10.1016/j.neubiorev.2012.02.007

[7] Brian J, Bryson SE, Garon N, Roberts W, Smith IM, Szatmari P, et al. Clinical assessment of autism in high-risk 18-month- olds. Autism: The International Journal of Research and Practice. 2008;**12**(5):433-456. DOI: 10.1177/1362361308094500

[8] Teitelbaum P, Teitelbaum O, Nye J, Fryman J, Maurer RG. Movement analysis in infancy may be useful for early diagnosis of autism. Proceedings of the National Academy of Sciences of the United States of America. 1998;**95**(23):13982-13987. DOI: 10.1073/pnas.95.23.13982

[9] Fournier KA, Kimberg CI, Radonovich KJ, Tillman MD, Chow JW, Lewis MH, et al. Decreased static and dynamic postural control in children with autism spectrum disorders. Gait and Posture. 2010;**32**:6-9

[10] Lai MC, Lombardo MV, Baron-Cohen S. Autism. Lancet (London, England). 2014;**383**(9920):896-910. DOI: 10.1016/S0140-6736(13)61539-1

[11] Gong L, Liu Y, Yi L, Fang J, Yang U, Wei K. Abnor mal gait patterns in autism spectrum disorder and their correla tions with social impairments. Autism Research. 2020;**13**:1215-1226. DOI: 10.1002/aur.2302

[12] Nobile M, Perego P, Piccinini L, Mani E, Rossi A, Bellina M, et al. Further evidence of complex motor dysfunc tion in drug naïve children with autism using automatic motion analysis of gait. Autism. 2011;**15**(3):263-283. DOI: 10.1177/1362361309356929

[13] Rinehart N, McGinley J. Is motor dysfunction core to autism spectrum disorder? Developmental Medicine and Child Neurology. 2010;**52**(8):697. DOI: 10.1111/j.1469-8749.2010.03631.x

[14] Bäckström A, Johansson AM, Rudolfsson T, Rönnqvist L, von Hofsten C, Rosander K, et al. Motor planning and movement execution during goal-directed sequential manual

movements in 6-year-old children with autism spectrum disorder: A kinematic analysis. Research in Developmental Disabilities. 2021;**115**:104014. DOI: 10.1016/j.ridd.2021.104014

[15] Forti S, Valli A, Perego P, Nobile M, Crippa A, Molteni M. Motor planning and control in autism a kinematic analysis of preschool children. Research in Autism Spectrum Disorders. 2011;**5**(2):834-842. DOI: 10.1016/j.rasd.2010.09.013

[16] Crippa A, Forti S, Perego P, Molteni M. Eye-hand coor dination in children with high functioning autism and Asperger's disorder using a gap-overlap paradigm. Journal of Autism and Developmental Disorders. 2013;**43**(4):841-850. DOI: 10.1007/s10803-012-1623-8

[17] Koegel LK, Koegel RL, Ashbaugh K, Bradshaw J. The importance of early identification and intervention for children with or at risk for autism spectrum disorders. International Journal of Speech-Language Pathology. 2014;**16**(1):50-56. DOI: 10.3109/17549507.2013.861511

[18] Lord C, Risi S, Lambrecht L, Cook EH Jr, Leventhal BL, DiLavore PC, et al. The autism diagnostic observation schedule-generic: A standard measure of social and communication deficits associated with the spectrum of autism. Journal of Autism and Developmental Disorders. 2000;**30**(3):205-223

[19] Perego P, Forti S, Crippa A, Valli A, Reni G. Reach and throw movement analysis with support vector machines in early diagnosis of autism. In: Annual International Conference of the IEEE Engineering in Medicine and Biology Society. IEEE Engineering in Medicine and Biology Society. Annual Interna Tional Conference, 2009. 2009. pp. 2555-2558. DOI: 10.1109/IEMBS.2009.5335096

[20] Vabalas A, Gowen E, Poliakoff E, Casson AJ. Kinematic features of a simple and short movement task to predict autism diagnosis. In: Annual International Conference of the IEEE Engineering in Medicine and Biology Society. IEEE Engineering in Medicine and Biology Society. Annual International Conference, 2019. 2019. pp. 1421-1424. DOI: 10.1109/EMBC.2019.8857307

[21] Milano N, Simeoli R, Rega A, Marocco D. A deep learning latent variable model to identify children with autism through motor abnormalities. Frontiers in Psychology. 2023;**14**:1194760. DOI: 10.3389/fpsyg.2023.1194760

[22] Sarker IH. Machine learning: Algorithms, real-world applications and research directions. SN Computer Science. 2021;**2**(3):160. DOI: 10.1007/s42979-021-00592-x

[23] von Hofsten C, Rosander K. Perception-action in children with ASD. Frontiers in Integrative Neuroscience. 2012;**6**:115. DOI: 10.3389/fnint.2012.00115

[24] Emanuele M, Nazzaro G, Marini M, Veronesi C, Boni S, Polletta G, et al. Motor synergies: Evidence for a novel motor signature in autism spectrum disorder. Cognition. 2021;**213**:104652. DOI: 10.1016/j.cogni tion.2021.104652

[25] Cavallo A, Romeo L, Ansuini C, Battaglia F, Nobili L, Pontil M, et al. Identifying the signature of prospective motor control in children with autism. Scientific Reports. 2021;**11**(1):3165. DOI: 10.1038/s41598-021-82374-2

[26] Crippa A, Salvatore C, Perego P, Forti S, Nobile M, Molteni M, et al.

Use of machine learning to identify children with autism and their motor abnormalities. Journal of Autism and Developmental Disorders. 2015;**45**(7):2146-2156. DOI: 10.1007/s10803-015-2379-8

[27] Vabalas A, Gowen E, Poliakoff E, Casson AJ. Applying machine learning to kinematic and eye movement features of a movement imitation task to predict autism diagnosis. Science Reports. 2020;**10**:1-13. DOI: 10.1038/s41598-020-65384-4

[28] Li B, Sharma A, Meng J, Purushwalkam S, Gowen E. Applying machine learning to identify autistic adults using imitation: An exploratory study. PLoS One. 2017;**12**(8):e0182652. DOI: 10.1371/journal.pone.0182652

[29] Anzulewicz A, Sobota K, Delafield-Butt JT. Toward the autism motor signature: Gesture patterns during smart tablet gameplay identify children with autism. Science Reports. 2016;**6**:1-13. DOI: 10.1038/srep31107

[30] Simeoli R, Milano N, Rega A, Marocco D. Using technology to identify children with autism through motor abnormalities. Frontiers in Psychology. 2021;**12**:635696. DOI: 10.3389/fpsyg.2021.635696

[31] Raya MA, Giglioli IA, Marín-Morales J, Higuera-Trujillo JL, Olmos E, Minissi ME, et al. Application of supervised machine learning for behavioral biomarkers of autism spectrum disorder based on electrodermal activity and virtual reality. Frontiers in Human Neuroscience. 2020b;**14**:90. DOI: 10.3389/fnhum.2020.00090

[32] Alcañiz Raya M, Marín-Morales J, Minissi ME, Teruel Garcia G, Abad L, Chicchi Giglioli IA. Machine learning and virtual reality on body movements' behaviors to classify children with autism spectrum disorder. Journal of Clinical Medicine. 2020;**9**(5):1260. DOI: 10.3390/jcm9051260

[33] Robles M, Namdarian N, Otto J, Wassiljew E, Navab N, Falter Wagner C, et al. A virtual reality based system for the screening and classification of autism. IEEE Transactions on Visualization and Computer Graphics. 2022;**28**(5):2168-2178. DOI: 10.1109/TVCG.2022.3150489

[34] Kojovic N, Natraj S, Mohanty SP, Maillart T, Schaer M. Using 2D video-based pose estimation for automated prediction of autism spectrum disorders in young children. Scientific Reports. 2021;**11**(1):15069. DOI: 10.1038/s41598-021-94378-z

[35] Zhao Z, Zhu Z, Zhang X, Tang H, Xing J, Hu X, et al. Identifying autism with head movement features by implementing machine learning algorithms. Journal of Autism and Developmental Disorders. 2022;**52**(7):3038-3049. DOI: 10.1007/s10803-021-05179-2

[36] Li Y, Mache MA, Todd TA. Automated identification of postural control for children with autism spectrum disorder using a machine learning approach. Journal of Biomechanics. 2020;**113**:110073. DOI: 10.1016/j.jbiomech.2020.110073

[37] Frazier TW, Strauss M, Klingemier EW, Zetzer EE, Hardan AY, Eng C, et al. A meta-analysis of gaze differences to social and nonsocial information between individuals with and without autism. Journal of the American Academy of Child and Adolescent Psychiatry. 2017;**56**(7):546-555. DOI: 10.1016/j.jaac.2017.05.005

[38] Liu W, Li M, Yi L. Identifying children with autism spectrum disorder based on their face processing abnormality: A machine learning framework. Autism Research: Official Journal of the International Society for Autism Research. 2016;**9**(8):888-898. DOI: 10.1002/aur.1615

[39] Jiang M, Francis SM, Srishyla D, Conelea C, Zhao Q, Jacob S. Classifying individuals with ASD through facial emotion recognition and eye-tracking. In: Annual International Conference of the IEEE Engineering in Medicine and Biology Society. Annual International Conference. IEEE Engineering in Medicine and Biology Society; 2019. pp. 6063-6068. DOI: 10.1109/EMBC.2019.8857005

[40] Wan G, Kong X, Sun B, Yu S, Tu Y, Park J, et al. Applying eye tracking to identify autism spectrum disorder in children. Journal of Autism and Developmental Disorders. 2019;**49**(1):209-215. DOI: 10.1007/s10803-018-3690-y

[41] Liaqat S, Wu C, Duggirala PR, Cheung SS, Chuah CN, Ozonoff S, et al. Predicting ASD diagnosis in children with synthetic and image-based eye gaze data. Signal Processing. Image Communication. 2021;**94**:116198. DOI: 10.1016/j.image. 2021.116198

[42] Alcañiz M, Chicchi-Giglioli IA, Carrasco-Ribelles LA, Marín Morales J, Minissi ME, Teruel-García G, et al. Eye gaze as a biomarker in the recognition of autism spectrum disorder using virtual reality and machine learning: A proof of concept for diagnosis. Autism Research: Official Journal of the International Society for Autism Research. 2022;**15**(1):131-145. DOI: 10.1002/aur.2636

[43] Elbattah M, Carette R, Dequen G, Guérin J-L, Cilia F. Learning clusters in autism spectrum disorder: Image-based clustering of eye-tracking scanpaths with deep autoencoder. In: 2019 41st Annual International Conference of the IEEE Engineering in Medicine and Biology Society (EMBC). 2019. pp. 1417-1420. DOI: 10.1109/EMBC.2019.8856904

[44] Tsuchiya KJ, Hakoshima S, Hara T, Ninomiya M, Saito M, Fujioka T, et al. Diagnosing autism spectrum disorder without expertise: A pilot study of 5- to 17-year-old individuals using Gazefinder. Frontiers in Neurology. 2021;**11**:603085. DOI: 10.3389/fneur.2020.603085

[45] Cilia F, Carette R, Elbattah M, Dequen G, Guérin JL, Bosche J, et al. Computer-aided screening of autism spectrum disorder: Eye-tracking study using data visualization and deep learning. JMIR Human Factors. 2021;**8**(4):e27706. DOI: 10.2196/27706

[46] Kanhirakadavath MR, Chandran MSM. Investigation of eye-tracking scan path as a biomarker for autism screening using machine learning algorithms. Diagnostics (Basel, Switzerland). 2022;**12**(2):518. DOI: 10.3390/diagnostics12020518

[47] Lin Y, Gu Y, Xu Y, Hou S, Ding R, Ni S. Autistic spectrum traits detection and early screening a machine learning based eye movement study. Journal of Child and Adolescent Psychiatric Nursing Official Publication of the Association of Child and Adolescent Psychiatric Nurses Inc. 2022;**35**(1):83-92. DOI: 10.1111/jcap.12346

[48] De Jaegher H. Embodiment and sense-making in autism. Frontiers in Integrative Neuroscience. 2013;**7**:15. DOI: 10.3389/fnint.2013.00015

[49] Hyde KK, Novack MN, LaHaye N, Parlett-Pelleriti C, Anden R, Dixon DR,

et al. Applications of supervised machine learning in autism spectrum disorder research: A review. Review Journal of Autism and Developmental Disorders. 2019;**6**:128-146. DOI: 10.1007/s40489-019-00158-x

[50] Vabalas A, Freeth M. Brief report: Patterns of eye movements in face to face conversation are associated with autistic traits: Evidence from a student sample. Journal of Autism and Developmental Disorders. 2016;**46**(1):305-314. DOI: 10.1007/s10803-015-2546-y

[51] Pierce K, Carter C, Weinfeld M, Desmond J, Hazin R, Bjork R, et al. Detecting, studying, and treating autism early: The one-year well-baby check-up approach. The Journal of Pediatrics. 2011;**159**(3):458-465.e4656. DOI: 10.1016/j.jpeds.2011.02.036

[52] Cook JL, Blakemore SJ, Press C. Atypical basic movement kinematics in autism spectrum conditions. Brain. 2013;**136**:2816-2824. DOI: 10.1093/brain/awt208

[53] Torres EB, Brincker M, Isenhower RW, Yanovich P, Stigler KA, Nurnberger JI, et al. Autism: The micro movement perspective. Frontiers in Integrative Neuroscience. 2013;7:32. DOI: 10.3389/fnint.2013.00032

[54] Whyatt C, Craig CM. Interceptive skills in children aged 9-11 years, diagnosed with autism spectrum disorder. Research in Autism Spectrum Disorder. 2013;7:613-623. DOI: 10.1016/j.rasd.2013.01.003

[55] Klin A, Jones W, Schultz R, Volkmar F. The enactive mind, or from actions to cognition: Lessons from autism. Philosophical Transactions of the Royal Society of London. Series B, Biological Sciences. 2003;**358**:345-360. DOI: 10.1098/rstb.2002.1202

[56] Fabbri-Destro M, Cattaneo L, Boria S, Rizzolatti G. Planning actions in autism. Experimental Brain Research. 2009;**192**:521-525. DOI: 10.1007/s00221-008-1578-3

[57] Trevarthen C, Delafield-Butt JT. Autism as a developmental disorder in intentional movement and affective engagement. Frontiers in Integrative Neuroscience. 2013;7:49. DOI: 10.3389/fnint.2013.00049

[58] Mari M, Castiello U, Marks D, Marraffa C, Prior M. The reach-to grasp movement in children with autism spectrum disorder. Philosophical Transactions of the Royal Society B. 2003;**358**:393-403. DOI: 10.1098/rstb.2002.1205

[59] Papadopoulos N, McGinley J, Tonge BJ, Bradshaw JL, Saunders K, Rinehart NJ. An investigation of upper limb motor function in high functioning autism and Asperger's disorder using a repetitive Fitts' aiming task. Research in Autism Spectrum Disorder. 2012;**6**:286-292. DOI: 10.1016/j.rasd.2011.05.010

[60] Pierno AC, Mari M, Glover S, Georgiou I, Castiello U. Failure to read motor intentions from gaze in children with autism. Neuropsychologia. 2006;**44**:1483-1488. DOI: 10.1016/j.neuropsychologia.2005.11.013

[61] Cattaneo L, Fabbri-Destro M, Boria S, Pieraccini C, Monti A, Cossu G, et al. Impairment of actions chains in autism and its possible role in intention understanding. Proceedings. National Academy of Sciences. United States of America. 2007;**104**:17825-17830. DOI: 10.1073/pnas.0706273104

Chapter 3

# The Role of Copy Number Variations in Autism Spectrum Disorders and Genetic Approaches

*Nagehan Bilgeç*

## Abstract

Autism Spectrum Disorder (ASD) is the most common neurodevelopmental disorder in children, characterised by restricted and repetitive behaviours and interests, challenging social interaction and communication. ASD is a complicated condition shaped by a combination of genetic, epigenetic, and environmental factors, but genetics play a crucial role in its aetiology. Numerous studies have demonstrated that genetic factors significantly contribute to the development of autism. Although there are clinically identifiable syndromes and molecularly identifiable syndromes in autism, a significant number remain for which we have yet to elucidate the genetic cause. Chromosomal abnormalities, microdeletion syndromes, and single-gene disorders constitute the foundation of the genetic disorders that result in autism. While the success rate in determining a specific etiological diagnosis in patients with ASD was reported as 6–15% in previous years, nowadays, genetic aetiology can be detected in approximately 40%. The rate of genetic diagnosis has increased with chromosomal microarray analysis and next-generation sequencing methods. Copy number variations (CNVs) cause clinical manifestation in patients as a result of haploinsufficiency and triplosensitivity of protein-coding genes and noncoding genes. Especially, protein-coding and noncoding genes, which are highly expressed in the brain, influence the regulation of neural stem cell differentiation, synaptic plasticity, axon guidance, and cortical development through their effects on gene expression. In this way, protein-coding and noncoding genes contribute to neuropsychiatric and neurodevelopmental disorders. Detecting CNVs is crucial for understanding gene functions and interactions.

**Keywords:** Autism Spectrum Disorder, copy number variant, genetic testing, genetic factors, microarray-based comparative genomic hybridisation, array CGH, SNParray

## 1. Introduction

Autism was first defined by Leo Kanner in 1943 as a stereotyped behavioural pattern with restricted social and emotional communication in early childhood [1]. It was last defined as "Autism Spectrum Disorder" (ASD) by the American Psychiatric

 IntechOpen

Association and the World Health Organization in 2013, according to the DSM-5 diagnostic criteria [2]. ASD is the most common neurodevelopmental disorder in children, characterised by restricted and repetitive behaviours and interests, challenging social interaction and communication, beginning in the early developmental period before the age of 3 [3]. The prevalence of ASD is 1 in 36 children, which is seen in all socioeconomic and ethnic groups and varies among societies. ASD male-to-female ratio is nearly 4 [4].

Kanner emphasised that autism is potentially a congenital disorder but that the characteristic behavioural characteristics of the parents also affect the disease [1]. Asperger assumes that ASD tends to be transmitted from parent to child [5]. Bruno Bettelheim supported Kanner's perspective that autism emerges from the dynamics of the mother-child relationship, describing the term as "refrigerator mother" [6]. In the 1970s, Rutter et al. hypothesised that autism was a congenital cognitive impairment caused by substantial genetic factors. In a twin study by Folstein and Rutter, 21 twin pairs were examined, and it was reported that the concordance rate for autism among monozygotic twins was 36–82% when broader phenotypes were considered. In contrast, using the pairwise method, the concordance rate for dizygotic twins was 0%, increasing only to 10% when broader phenotypes were taken into account [7]. This striking difference underscores the significant genetic factors at play in the development of autism.

Autism Spectrum Disorder (ASD) is a complicated condition shaped by a combination of genetic, epigenetic, and environmental factors, but genetics play a crucial role in its aetiology [3]. Research, including population, family, and twin studies, demonstrates that ASD has a hereditary component. Theoretically, monozygotic (MZ) twins have an identical genetic makeup, sharing 100% of their inherited genetic material and environmental influences. However, this perfect ratio can be subject to slight variations. These differences often arise from epigenetic modifications, which can change gene expression without altering the DNA sequence, or postzygotic mitotic de novo mutations, which are spontaneous genetic changes that occur after the fertilisation of the egg. These factors illustrate the complexities of genetic similarity and how environmental interactions can shape the development of MZ twins over time [8]. A meta-analysis published in 2016 found that the concordance rate for MZ twin pairs was 98%, while the rate for dizygotic (DZ) twins was 53% [9]. When considering all twin study data, the consistency rate for ASD is approximately 45% for MZ twins and 16% for DZ twins [10]. In family studies, a large epidemiological study on autism conducted in Utah in the 1980s reported an 8.6% recurrence risk in siblings born after an affected child [11]. A study of 2920 children from 1235 families revealed that the probability of a sibling developing ASD if another sibling has the disorder is 10.9%. The incidence of a sibling having a history of "language delay or speech problems" was reported at 20%, while a risk of 14.2% was noted for siblings born later [12]. Furthermore, Ozonoff et al. indicated a familial recurrence rate of 20.2% among 1605 individuals with ASD from 18 international Baby Siblings Research Consortium sites [13]. The three-hit hypothesis proposes that three main factors influence the development of neurodevelopmental disorders. The first is a genetic predisposition; the second aspect clearly demonstrates that stress is influenced by the hypothalamic-pituitary-adrenal (HPA) axis and the autonomic nervous system, emphasising the critical role these systems play in our physiological responses to stress in early life, which affects critical periods of brain development. The last factor is late environmental influences, which are also linked to neurodevelopmental disorders through epigenetic mechanisms [14]. These findings indicate that environmental factors shape neurodevelopmental disorders based on genetic factors and that genetic factors have a considerable effect on the development of ASD.

## 2. Genetic classification of ASD

Research has identified several monogenic factors associated with ASD. The genetic causes of ASD include large chromosomal rearrangements, numerical and structural chromosomal abnormalities, changes in DNA sequence copy numbers and single-nucleotide variants (SNVs). When ASD occurs alongside a clinically defined pattern of congenital anomalies, it is referred to as syndromic autism. Various chromosomal abnormalities and microdeletion syndromes, as well as triplet repeat disorders like Fragile X Syndrome, single-gene disorders such as Tuberous Sclerosis, PTEN-associated macrocephaly-autism syndrome and Rett Syndrome, play a significant role in a substantial number of ASD cases with identified genetic origins. Additionally, very rarely, metabolic disorders such as mitochondrial disorders and Sanfilippo syndrome are involved. In contrast, the isolated neurobehavioural phenotype without a known genetic cause is termed idiopathic autism [15]. In particular, CNVs are found in 10–20% of individuals with ASD, and 3% are large CNVs that cytogenetic methods can detect. The emergence of chromosomal microarray and next-generation sequencing techniques has revealed a wide range of CNVs associated with ASD [3]. Basically, we can divide ASD genetically into three groups: clinically identifiable syndromes, molecularly identifiable syndromes and unknown group (**Figure 1**).

There is a relationship between gene dosage changes and autism associated with numerical chromosomal abnormalities. In addition to multiple congenital anomalies that come with trisomies, the incidence of ASD is also elevated. Specifically, the incidence of ASD in individuals with trisomy 21 is 37.7% [16]. Similarly, the prevalence of autism is higher in individuals with sex chromosome aneuploidies. For instance, the prevalence of autism in individuals with XYY trisomy is approximately 30%, XXY trisomy is approximately 25%, and XXX trisomy is about 15% [17]. A study by Berry et al. found that 45X aneuploidy had the most significant impact on ASD risk, followed by 47XYY, 47 XXY and 47XXX aneuploidies in a large case-control study on ASD [18].

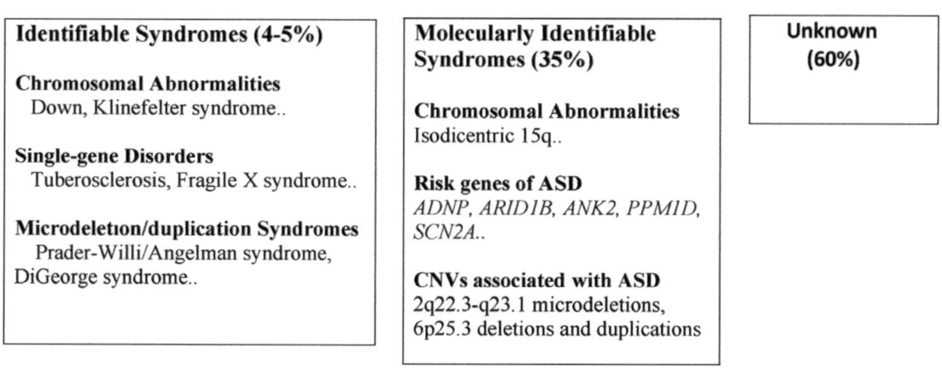


**Figure 1.**
*Schematic representation of the genetic classification of Autism Spectrum Disorder (ASD).*

Copy number variations (CNVs) are common and constitute 4.8–9.5% of the human genome [19]. The majority of the individuals, approximately 95%, is considered common variants, which are thought to contribute to genetic diversity. Around 1% of CNVs are classified as rare variants and may be crucial in the genetic basis of various neurodevelopmental disorders, including autism [20]. Denovo CNVs are present in about 10% of individuals diagnosed with simplex autism and 3% of families affected by multiplex autism. This contrasts with the 1–2% of unaffected siblings and control groups [3, 21].

## 3. Genetic studies

Direct genetic testing may be requested to assess syndromic patients with a preliminary diagnosis. For clinically recognised chromosomal aneuploidies such as Down syndrome and Klinefelter syndrome, conventional cytogenetic studies are recommended. Techniques such as fluorescence in situ hybridisation or multiplex ligation-dependent probe amplification are preferred in cases involving recognised microdeletion syndromes. Targeted single-gene sequencing or next-generation sequencing (NGS) panels are the most appropriate options for single-gene disorders. Conducting a comprehensive clinical evaluation of the patient and a referral to a clinical geneticist is essential. First, a detailed patient history should be taken, a three-generation pedigree should be drawn, and the patient should be evaluated with a detailed physical examination. If an additional finding leads to a specific diagnosis, tests directed to it should be continued in the diagnostic algorithm. In instances of idiopathic autism, submicroscopic CNVs and single nucleotide variants (SNVs) or insertions/deletions (indels) have been reported. Diagnosis often involves microarray-based comparative genomic hybridisation (array CGH), single nucleotide polymorphism (SNP) arrays and CNV analysis based on sequencing, particularly with advancements provided by next-generation sequencing (NGS) technologies.

CNVs range from 50 bp to 3 Mb, while smaller elements are called indels [22]. Array CGH detects chromosomal microdeletions and microduplications, while chromosomal SNP microarray analysis identifies abnormalities 100 times smaller than those detected by high-resolution chromosome methods. An array's resolution and diagnostic rate are directly influenced by the types, size and number of probes used and their distribution throughout the genome. In general, a higher number of probes with better uniformity in the array contribute to increased sensitivity. Due to the microarrays having limitations in detecting small-scale CNVs, the use of NGS allows us to detect small-scale CNVs [3]. Array CGH technology is a fast method for detecting the association between CNVs and Autism Spectrum Disorder (ASD) risks [20].

The assumed role of CNVs is likely related to their position in the genome, and their effects vary depending on whether they cause haploinsufficiency or triinsufficiency in the gene. The detected CNVs are examined using collaborative databases, including the Clinical Genomic Resource (ClinGen) (http://clinicalgenome.org/), the Database of Chromosomal Imbalance and Phenotype in Humans Using Ensembl Resources (Decipher) (http://decipher.sanger.ac.uk/), (Simons Foundation Autism Research Initiative [SFARI, https://www.sfari.org/resource/sfari-gene/], the European Cytogeneticists Association's Register of Unbalanced Chromosome Aberrations (ECARUCA) (http://umcecaruca01.extern.umcn.nl:8080/ecaruca/ecaruca.jsp), the Ensembl Genome Browser (http://www.ensembl.org/index.html), the National Center for Biotechnology Information (NCBI) (http://www.ncbi.nlm.nih.gov/) and the University California Santa Cruz (UCSC) Genome Browser (http://

genome.ucsc.edu/) for evaluation of pathogenicity. CNVs were classified as pathogenic, likely pathogenic, variant of unknown significance, likely benign and benign according to the American College of Medical Genetics and Genomics guideline [22]. The features of genes described in CNVs, such as phenotypes, disorders, sequence paralogs, expression patterns and gene ontology, are evaluated using Genecards and GeneDecks (http://www.genecards.org/index.php?path=/GeneDecks).

Syndromic autism accounts for about 15% of cases, while idiopathic autism makes up approximately 85% [15]. Patients diagnosed with autism who lack a positive family history are referred to as having simplex autism, while individuals with a first-degree relative with autism are classified as multiplex autism [3]. CNVs are linked to 5–10% of simplex ASD cases and 2–3% of ASD patients from multiplex families [23]. Since 2010, the International Standards for Cytogenomic Arrays (ISCA) Consortium has strongly endorsed chromosomal microarray as the essential initial diagnostic assessment for children with ASD and various developmental disorders [24]. Multiple studies confirm the effective diagnostic yield of aCGH, revealing that clinically relevant CNVs are found in 9.3–29.0% of patients with idiopathic autism [25].

Exome sequencing is a method that sequences exonic and exon-intron junction regions in the genome. Recently, with the advent of NGS technologies, CNV based on sequencing analysis has been used to detect both SNV/indels and CNVs in neurodevelopmental disorders. Many studies have examined the diagnostic yield. Miyake et al. detected the diagnostic yield of pathogenic SNVs and indels at 13.1% (53 individuals) and CNVs at 3.2% (13 individuals) by CNV based on exome sequencing among 405 individuals with ASD. In this study, the diagnostic yield of simplex families was 17.7%, (62/351), whereas it was 7.4% for multiplex families (4/54) [26]. Feliciano et al. detected that the diagnostic yield in multiplex families was 15.2% and in simplex families was 10.1%. This data were obtained from whole exome sequencing (WES) applied to 457 families with ASD, consisting of 418 simplex and 39 multiplex families. This study found 647 rare de novo SNVs and indels in coding regions and splice sites [27]. The diagnostic yield of ASD using array CGH analyses is reported to be between 3.0% and 9.3%, while the yield using exome sequencing (ES) ranges from 6.1% to 8.4% [26]. Recent studies demonstrate that WES can provide a diagnostic yield of 35% for individuals with intellectual disabilities and global developmental delay and 15% for individuals diagnosed with ASD [28].

CNVs cause clinical manifestation in patients as a result of haploinsufficiency and triplosensitivity of protein-coding genes and noncoding genes. Long noncoding RNA (lncRNA) are longer than 200 nucleotides that do not code for proteins but play key regulatory roles in biological processes [29]. LncRNAs make gene regulation and chromatin remodelling and regulate miRNA-mRNA and protein-protein interactions, affecting gene expression epigenetically, transcriptionally and post-transcriptionally. LncRNAs are highly expressed in the brain and regulate neural stem cell differentiation, synaptic plasticity, axon guidance and cortical development with their effects on gene expression [30]. In this way, many lncRNAs have been associated with ASD. Variations of both protein-coding genes and noncoding genes disrupt neurodevelopmental pathways, leading to neurodevelopmental disorders. Abedini et al. associated 1632 genes with ASD, including both protein-coding genes and long noncoding RNAs, within the 47 CNV regions. The coding genes and lncRNA genes located within the CNV region are crucial players in the development of neurodevelopmental disorders and ASD, highlighting the importance of this genetic region in understanding these complex conditions [31]. Numerous coding genes and lncRNA genes within the CNV region play a significant role in neurodevelopmental disorders (NDD) and Autism Spectrum Disorder (ASD). The genes strongly linked to autism are listed in **Table 1** [31–35].

| Microarray region | Deletion | Coding genes in the region | lncRNA genes in the region |
|---|---|---|---|
| 1p36 | del | *DVL1, DNAJC11, VWA1, GNB1, PRKCZ, RERE*[31] *GABRD*[32] *SPEN*[33] | *RP11-206 L10, TP73-AS1, CATG00000045106, CATG00000004170, CATG00000004816, CATG00000004823*[31] |
| 1q21.1 | dup | *BCL9*[31] | *RP11–337C18*[31] |
| 1q41 | del | | *DISP1, SUSD4, FBXO28, TP53BP2 WDR26*[34] |
| 2p16.3 | del | *NRXN1*[31] | *AC007682.1*[31] |
| 2q23.1 | del | *MBD5, ACVR2A*[31] | |
| 2q37 | del | | *AC131097.3, AC093642.3, AC093642*[31] |
| 3q29 | del | *FBXO45, PAK2, DLG1*[31] | *CATG00000067412, MFI2-AS1, AC128709.2*[31] |
| 4q16.3 | del | | *FGFR3, NAT8L*[31] |
| 6p25.3 | del/dup | | *DUSP22*[31] |
| 7q11.23 | | *STX1A, GTF2I, CLIP2, FZD9, LIMK1, EIF4H, GTF2IRD1*[31] | *CATG00000096069, CATG00000092613, CATG00000096089*[31] |
| 8p23.1 | del/dup | | *TNKS, PINX1, MSRA, XKR6, FAM167A, NEIL2, RP11–1E4.1*[31] |
| 9q34.3 | del | | *EHMT1, CACNA1B*[31] |
| 10q22-q23 | del | | *GRID1, BMPR1A, NRG3*[31] |
| 11p14.1-p13 | del | | *KCNA4, ELP4*[31] |
| 13q34 | del | | *MCF2L, UPF3A*[35] |
| 15q11.2-q13.3 | del/dup | *UBE3A, GABRB3, GABRA5, GABRG3, HERC2, APBA2, NIPA1, ARHGAP11B, FAN1, TRPM1, CHRNA7*[31] | *CATG00000024385, RP11–484P15, CATG00000022353, CATG00000022386, CATG00000024462, CATG00000022467*[31] |
| 16p11.2-p13.11 16p12.2 | | *KCTD13, PRRT2, SEZ6L2, DOC2A, TBX6, MAPK3, SH2B1*[31] | *CATG00000028919, CATG00000028920*[31] |
| 17p11.2-p13.3 | del/dup | *ASPA, TRPV1, RTN4RL1 YWHAE, RASD1, RAI1, PAFAH1B1*[31] | *CATG00000030828, CATG00000032809, RP11– 74E22.3, CATG00000030472, CATG00000032796, CATG00000032809*[31] |
| 17q21.31 | del | *RP11–445F12, RP11– 697E22, MAPT-AS1*[31] | *LHX1, CRHR1, MAPT, KANSL1*[31] |
| 18q21 | del | *TCF4*[36] | |
| 21q11.2 | del | *CRKL, RTN4R, ZDHHC8, SEPT5, MAPK1, GNAZ, BCR*[31] | *XXbac-B444P24.14, DGCR5, AC000068.5, CATG00000058233, CATG00000058251, LL22NC03–86G*[31] |
| 21q11.2 | dup | *RTN4R, ZDHHC8, SEPT5*[31] | *XXbac-B444P24.14, AC000068.5*[31] |
| 22q13.2 | del | *SHANK3, MAPK8IP2, TTLL1, MLC1, BRD1, PANX2, MAPK11, PLXNB2*[31] | *CATG00000057830, RP3–388 M5, CTA-217C2, CATG00000057926, RP3–402G11.26, CHKBAS1, CATG00000058090, CATG00000058095*[31] |
| Xp22.31 deletion | del | *PNPLA4, STS*[31] | |
| Xp22.33 | dup | *ASMT, ASMTL-AS1*[31] | *CATG00000112948*[31] |

**Table 1.**
*Coding genes and lncRNA genes in the CNV region which play a major role NDDs and ASD.*

In this section, contiguous gene syndromes associated with ASD and their features will be discussed.

## 4. Contiguous gene syndromes

### 4.1 Wolf-Hirschhorn syndrome (chromosome 4p16.3 deletion syndrome)

Wolf-Hirschhorn Syndrome (WHS) results from a partial loss of the distal portion of the short (p) arm of chromosome 4 (4p16.3). The size of this loss varies, reflecting the spectrum and severity of the disease. Most cases are due to a de novo deletion of chromosome 4p. In 20% of cases, an unbalanced translocation involving chromosome 4 in the parental karyotype can lead to deletion. Complex genomic rearrangements, including ring 4 chromosomes, are present in fewer cases. Characteristic clinical points of WHS, including prenatal and postnatal growth deficiency, distinctive facial features consisting of 'Greek warrior helmet' appearance, intellectual disability (ID), hypotonia, epilepsy or EEG anomalies, a large variety of skeletal anomalies (split hand; talipes equinovarus, scoliosis), congenital cardiac defects and genito-urinary tract defects (vesicoureteral reflux, horseshoe kidney, uni/bilateral renal agenesis, cystic dysplasia/ hypoplasia, and oligomeganephroma, uni/bilateral cryptorchidism, in males, and clitoral aplasia/hyperplasia, streak gonads, and absent uterus/vagina), are seen [36]. Cognitive deficits ranging from mild to severe were seen in all patients, while attention deficit disorder, attention-deficit/hyperactivity disorder (ADHD) and ASD were reported [37, 38].

### 4.2 Williams-Beuren syndrome (chromosome 7q11.23 deletion syndrome)

Williams-Beuren Syndrome (WS) results from a de novo 1.5- to 1.8-Mb 7q11.23 deletion; an individual with WS rarely has an affected parent. WS is characterised by developmental delay, mild to moderate ID, unique personality, distinctive facies (broad forehead, bitemporal narrowing, periorbital fullness, a stellate/lacy iris pattern, strabismus, short nose, broad nasal tip, wide mouth, long philtrum, thick vermilion of the upper and lower lips, malocclusion, small jaw, and large ear lobes), cardiovascular disease (supravalvar aortic stenosis, peripheral pulmonary stenosis, hypertension), connective tissue abnormalities (hyperextensible joints, hyperlaxity), endocrine abnormalities (hypercalcemia, hypercalciuria, hypothyroidism, early puberty), feeding difficulties in infancy, and obesity in childhood [39]. The characteristic personality profile of WS includes overfriendliness, social disinhibition, excessive empathy, attention problems and non-social anxiety. ASD is seen in 10–20% of cases, as well as restricted interests and repetitive behaviour [40].

### 4.3 Prader-Willi syndrome

Prader-Willi Syndrome (PWS) results from the absence of a paternally expressed imprinted genes. Approximately 70% of cases have paternal 15q11-q13 deletion, 20–30% of cases have abnormal DNA methylation within the Prader-Willi critical region (PWCR) at 15q11-q13 due to maternal uniparental disomy (UPD), 2.5% of cases have an imprinting center mutation at PWCR. PWS presents with severe hypotonia, poor appetite and feeding difficulties in early infancy, followed in early childhood by excessive eating and obesity, short stature, small hands and feet, distinctive facial appearance (bitemporal narrowing, almond-shaped eyes, strabismus, upslanting palpebral fissure, small mouth, thin upper lip, down-turned corners of the mouth) hypogonadism, ID and behavioural abnormalities [41]. A characteristic behaviour profile with anxiety, temper tantrums, self-injurious, rigidity/resistance to change, obsessive-compulsive behaviours, ADHD and social cognition deficits becomes evident in early childhood in individuals with PWS. These behaviours and psychosis increase with age in adolescence [42].

ASD is seen in approximately 26.7% of those with PWS, and the frequency of ASD is thought to be 35.3% in cases due to uniparental disomy, while it is 18.5% in cases due to deletion. It has been reported that the symptoms of PWS + ASD are fewer and milder in severity than IO [43].

### 4.4 Angelman syndrome

Angelman syndrome (AS) occurs due to maternal allele loss or lack of expression in the chromosome 15q11-q13 region [44]. Maternal 15q11-q13 deletion is responsible for 70% of the molecular mechanisms of aetiology. 10% of cases have maternally inherited UBE3A mutations. The rest is due to paternal UPD of chromosome 15q11-q13, imprinting defects that disrupt the expression of maternally inherited UBE3A [45].

AS is characterised by microcephaly and characteristic facial appearance (flat occiput, widely spaced teeth, wide mouth, protruding tongue, prognathia, light skin-hair-eyes); wide-based, ataxic gait; frequent laughter; smiling and excitability with a happy appearance; absent or impaired speech; developmental delay; ID and epilepsy [44]. All the molecular causes of AS result in a similar phenotype, which includes severe to profound ID, characteristic behavioural abnormalities and speech impairment. 50–81% of AS patients are diagnosed with ASD. Compared to patients with idiopathic autism, there is less impact on general developmental levels such as social smiling, enjoying mutual interaction and responding when called by name. The characteristic features of ASD, such as finger/hand movements, rotating objects and lining up objects, are rarely reported [46].

### 4.5 Chromosome 16p (16p11.2; 16p12.2; 16p13.11) deletion syndrome

The 16p region is an autism-susceptibility locus, and many duplications and deletions have been reported. Rearrangements within the 16p11.2 and 16p13.11 regions are associated with neurological disorders (seizures/epilepsy, ID, motor speech disorders) and neuropsychiatric disorders (autism, ADHD) [47].

The 16p11.2 deletion phenotype is characterised by motor coordination difficulties, motor speech disorder, speech impairment, psychiatric disorders, autistic features and severe early-onset obesity. Psychiatric diagnoses such as ADHD, autism, anxiety and obsessive-compulsive disorder, oppositional defiant disorder, conduct disorder and schizophrenia are present. 50% of individuals with a 16p11.2 deletion have ≥1 psychiatric/behavioural diagnosis. The most common are ADHD (%35) and autism (%25) [48]. 16p12.2 deletion syndrome is characterised by mild to profound ID, developmental delay, short stature, cardiac malformations, epilepsy, psychiatric/behavioural disorders, hearing loss, dental abnormalities, renal and genital anomalies and cleft palate ± cleft lip. Psychiatric and/or behavioural issues were identified in more than half of individuals with a 16p12.2 deletion [49]. The frequency of autism

*DOI: http://dx.doi.org/10.5772/intechopen.1010383*

has been reported as 46–67% [49, 50]. The 16p13.11 locus is an unstable genomic region with numerous low-copy number repeats. 16p13.1 is an extremely rare copy number variant. In the literature, it has been reported to clinically cause motor delay, facial dysmorphisms, microcephaly, gastroesophageal reflux disease (GERD), congenital heart defects, several neuropsychiatric conditions such as global developmental delay, psychiatric and behavioural problems and seizures and, less commonly, obesity [51].

### 4.6 Smith-Magenis syndrome (chromosome 17p11.2 deletion syndrome)

Smith-Magenis syndrome (SMS) is a neurodevelopmental disorder resulting from deletion or a pathogenic variant of the RAI1 gene located within the 17p11.2 region. SMS is characterised by distinctive physical features (broad square-shaped face, brachycephaly, prominent forehead, midface retrusion, synophrys, deep-set, hypertelorism, relative prognathism), developmental delay, ID, behavioural abnormalities, sleep disturbance, and childhood-onset abdominal obesity [52].

Most individuals have mild to moderate ID, sleep-wake disorders, stereotypies such as self-hugging/arm and/or hand-squeezing behaviours and self-injurious and physically aggressive behaviours; anxiety is common, and problems with executive functions such as inattention, distractibility, hyperactivity and impulsivity are also common. Self-harming stereotypic behaviours are found. Approximately 40% of the case studies reported features related to ASD and ADHD [53].

### 4.7 DiGeorge syndrome (chromosome 22q11.2 deletion syndrome)

22q11.2DS is caused by a 3.0 (2.54)-Mb deletion. More than 90% of cases occur de novo deletion, and about 10% are inherited from a heterozygous parent. Clinical features vary significantly, even among individuals from the same family. The most important clinical findings observed in these cases include palatal abnormalities (velopharyngeal insufficiency, cleft palate, bifid uvula), conotruncal malformations, immune deficiencies, characteristic facial features (hypertelorism, short palpebral fissures, low-set ears, prominent nasal bridge, micrognathia), sensorineural or conductive hearing loss, developmental delays and learning difficulties. It is well established that individuals with 22q11.2DS may exhibit behavioural disorders and a propensity for various psychiatric conditions. While impulse control disorders can occur, shyness and avoidant behaviours are also commonly reported. Attention deficit, anxiety and difficulties in social relationships are prevalent. The frequency of ASD is reported to be approximately 20% [54].

### 4.8 Phelan-McDermid syndrome-SHANK3 related (chromosome 22q13.3 deletion syndrome)

Phelan-McDermid syndrome-SHANK3 related (PMS-SHANK3 related) is caused by heterozygous deletion at chromosome 22q13.3 with involvement of at least part of SHANK3 or a heterozygous pathogenic variant in SHANK3. PMS-SHANK3 related is characterised by neonatal hypotonia, global developmental delay, physical dysmorphic features (microcephaly or macrocephaly, long eyelashes, pointed chin, broad nose, wide nasal bridge, bulbous nose, malocclusion, periorbital fullness, large, fleshy hands), ID, absent or impaired speech and autistic features. The neurobehavioural phenotype includes ASD, ADHD, aggressiveness towards others, irritability, habitual chewing or mouthing, tooth grinding, schizophrenia and bipolar disorder [55]. The neurobehavioural findings are typically caused by haploinsufficiency of the *SHANK3* gene, which plays a crucial role in forming and managing dendritic spines and excitatory synapses [56]. Approximately 65% of individuals with PMS are diagnosed with ASD [57].

## 5. Conclusion

A combination of genetic, epigenetic, and environmental factors plays a vital role in the development of ASD. Research involving twin studies has demonstrated the significant role that genetic factors play in the development of autism. The development of autism in the follow-up of monozygotic twins diagnosed with achondroplasia, who lack a family history of ASD, is unique in the world and further underscores the significance of genetic factors [58]. Due to the high prevalence of autism in society, it is essential to determine to what extent the detected SNVs, indels and CNVs affect individual and population risks. Both rare and common variants are believed to contribute to the pathomechanism of ASD. Common variants may explain the genetic contribution at the population level, whereas rare and/or de novo variants are more likely to explain ASD at the individual level [29]. Detecting CNVs allows us to investigate gene-gene and protein-protein interactions of coding and noncoding genes in this region. It helps us identify the strongest candidate genes associated with neuropsychiatric and neurodevelopmental phenotypes.

## Author details

Nagehan Bilgeç
Department of Pediatric Genetics, Faculty of Medicine, Necmettin Erbakan University, Konya, Turkey

*Address all correspondence to: drnkbilgec@gmail.com

## References

[1] Kanner L. Autistic disturbances of affective contact. Nervous Child. 1943;**2**(3):217-250

[2] American Psychiatric Association, editor. Diagnostic and Statistical Manual of Mental Disorders: DSM-5. 5th ed. American Psychiatric Association; 2013

[3] Genovese A, Butler MG. Clinical assessment, genetics, and treatment approaches in autism spectrum disorder. International Journal of Molecular Sciences. 2020;**21**:4726

[4] Prevalence and characteristics of autism spectrum disorder among children aged 8 years — Autism and developmental disabilities monitoring network, 11 Sites, United States, 2020. Surveillance Summaries/March 24. 2023;**72**(2):1-14

[5] Asperger H. Die 'autistischen psychopathen' im kindesalter. Archiv fur Psychiatrie und Nervenkrankheiten. 1944;**117**:76-136

[6] Mandy W, Lai MC. Annual research review: The role of the environment in the developmental psychopathology of autism spectrum condition. Journal of Child Psychology and Psychiatry. 2016;**57**(3):271-292. DOI: 10.1111/jcpp.12501 (burdan bruno yu bul)

[7] Folstein S, Rutter M. Genetic influences and infantile autism. Nature. 1997;**265**(5596):726-728. DOI: 10.1038/265726a0

[8] Imamura A, Morimoto Y, Ono S, Kurotaki N, Kanegae S, Yamamoto N, et al. Şizofreni ve otizm spektrum bozukluğunun genetik ve çevresel faktörleri: İkiz çalışmalarından elde edilen bilgiler. Journal of Neural Transmission. 2020;**127**:1501-1515. DOI: 10.1007/s00702-020-02188-w

[9] Tick B, Bolton P, Happé F, Rutter M, Rijsdijk F. Heritability of autism spectrum disorders: A meta-analysis of twin studies. Journal of Child Psychology and Psychiatry. 2016;**57**(5):585-595. DOI: 10.1111/jcpp.12499. Epub 2015 Dec 27

[10] Huguet G, Benabou M, Bourgeron T. The genetics of autism spectrum disorders. In: Sassone-Corsi P, Christen Y, editors. A Time for Metabolism and Hormones. Cham (CH): Springer; 2016

[11] Ritvo ER, Jorde LB, Mason-Brothers A, Freeman BJ, Pingree C, Jones MB, et al. The UCLA-University of Utah epidemiologic survey of autism: Recurrence risk estimates and genetic counseling. The American Journal of Psychiatry. 1989;**146**(8):1032-1036. DOI: 10.1176/ajp.146.8.1032

[12] Constantino JN, Zhang Y, Frazier T, Abbacchi AM, Law P. Sibling recurrence and the genetic epidemiology of autism. The American Journal of Psychiatry. 2010;**167**(11):1349-1356. DOI: 10.1176/appi.ajp.2010.09101470. Epub 2010 Oct 1

[13] Ozonoff S, Young GS, Bradshaw J, Charman T, Chawarska K, Iverson JM, et al. Familial recurrence of autism: Updates from the baby siblings research consortium. Pediatrics. 2024;**154**(2):e2023065297. DOI: 10.1542/peds.2023-065297

[14] Daskalakis NP, Bagot RC, Parker KJ, Vinkers CH, de Kloet ER. The three-hit concept of vulnerability and resilience: Toward understanding adaptation to early-life adversity

outcome. Psychoneuroendocrinology. 2013;**38**(9):1858-1873. DOI: 10.1016/j.psyneuen.2013.06.008. Epub 2013 Jul 7

[15] National Institute of Health (2019). About Autism. National Human Genome Research Institute. Available from: https://www.genome.gov/Genetic-Disorders/Autism [Accessed: May 2019]

[16] Warner G, Moss J, Smith P, Howlin P. Autism characteristics and behavioural disturbances in ~ 500 children with Down's syndrome in England and Wales. Autism Research. 2014;7(4):433-441. DOI: 10.1002/aur.1371. Epub 2014 Mar 24

[17] van Rijn S, Stockmann L, Borghgraef M, Bruining H, van Ravenswaaij-Arts C, Govaerts L, et al. The social behavioral phenotype in boys and girls with an extra X chromosome (Klinefelter syndrome and Trisomy X): A comparison with autism spectrum disorder. Journal of Autism and Developmental Disorders. 2014;**44**:310-320

[18] Berry ASF, Finucane BM, Myers SM, Walsh LK, Seibert JM, Martin CL, et al. A genome-first study of sex chromosome aneuploidies provides evidence of Y chromosome dosage effects on autism risk. Nature Communications. 2024;**15**(1):8897. DOI: 10.1038/s41467-024-53211-7

[19] Zarrei M, MacDonald JR, Merico D, Scherer SW. A copy number variation map of the human genome. Nature Reviews. Genetics. 2015;**16**(3):172-183. DOI: 10.1038/nrg3871. Epub 2015 Feb 3

[20] Chen CH, Chen HI, Chien WH, Li LH, Wu YY, Chiu YN, et al. High resolution analysis of rare copy number variants in patients with autism spectrum disorder from Taiwan. Scientific Reports. 2017;7:11919. DOI: 10.1038/s41598-017-12081-4

[21] Kereszturi É. Diversity and classification of genetic variations in autism spectrum disorder. International Journal of Molecular Sciences. 2023;**24**(23):16768. DOI: 10.3390/ijms242316768

[22] MacDonald JR, Ziman R, Yuen RK, Feuk L, Scherer SW. The database of genomic variants: A curated collection of structural variation in the human genome. Nucleic Acids Research. 2014;**42**(Database issue):D986-D992. DOI: 10.1093/nar/gkt958. Epub 2013 Oct 29

[23] Kearney HM, Thorland EC, Brown KK, Quintero-Rivera F, South ST. American College of Medical Genetics standards and guidelines for interpretation and reporting of postnatal constitutional copy number variants. Genetics in Medicine. 2011;**13**:680-685. DOI: 10.1097/GIM.0b013e3182217a3a

[24] Miller DT, Adam MP, Aradhya S, Biesecker LG, Brothman AR, Carter NP, et al. Consensus statement: Chromosomal microarray is a first-tier clinical diagnostic test for individuals with developmental disabilities or congenital anomalies. American Journal of Human Genetics. 2010;**86**(5):749-764

[25] Cucinotta F, Lintas C, Tomaiuolo P, Baccarin M, Picinelli C, Castronovo P, et al. Diagnostic yield and clinical impact of chromosomal microarray analysis in autism spectrum disorder. Molecular Genetics & Genomic Medicine. 2023;**11**(8):e2182. DOI: 10.1002/mgg3.2182. Epub 2023 Apr 25

[26] Miyake N, Tsurusaki Y, Fukai R, Kushima I, Okamoto N, Ohashi K, et al. Molecular diagnosis of 405 individuals with autism spectrum disorder. European Journal of Human Genetics. 2024;**32**(12):1551-1558. DOI: 10.1038/s41431-023-01335-7. Epub 2023

[27] Feliciano P, Zhou X, Astrovskaya I, Turner TN, Wang T, Brueggeman L, et al. Exome sequencing of 457 autism families recruited online provides evidence for autism risk genes. NPJ Genomic Medicine. 2019;**4**:19. DOI: 10.1038/s41525-019-0093-8

[28] Savatt JM, Myers SM. Genetic testing in neurodevelopmental disorders. Frontiers in Pediatrics. 2021;**9**:526779. DOI: 10.3389/fped.2021.526779

[29] Chodurska B, Kunej T. Long non-coding RNAs in humans: Classification, genomic organization and function. Noncoding RNA Research. 2025;**11**:313-327. DOI: 10.1016/j.ncrna.2025.01.004

[30] Rusconi F, Battaglioli E, Venturin M. Psychiatric disorders and lncRNAs: A synaptic match. International Journal of Molecular Sciences. 2020;**21**(9):3030. DOI: 10.3390/ijms21093030

[31] Abedini SS, Akhavantabasi S, Liang Y, Heng JI, Alizadehsani R, Dehzangi I, et al. A critical review of the impact of candidate copy number variants on autism spectrum disorder. Mutation Research, Reviews in Mutation Research. 2024;**794**:108509. DOI: 10.1016/j.mrrev.2024.108509. Epub 2024 Jul 6

[32] Windpassinger C, Kroisel PM, Wagner K, Petek E. The human gamma-aminobutyric acid A receptor delta (GABRD) gene: Molecular characterisation and tissue-specific expression. Gene. 2002;**292**(1-2):25-31. DOI: 10.1016/s0378-1119(02)00649-2

[33] Radio FC, Pang K, Ciolfi A, Levy MA, Hernández-García A, Pedace L, et al. SPEN haploinsufficiency causes a neurodevelopmental disorder overlapping proximal 1p36 deletion syndrome with an episignature of X chromosomes in females. American Journal of Human Genetics. 2021;**108**(3):502-516. DOI: 10.1016/j.ajhg.2021.01.015. Epub 2021 Feb 16

[34] Chen CP, Chern SR, Wu PS, Chen SW, Wu FT, Wang W. Molecular cytogenetic characterization of a de novo chromosome 1q41-q42.11 microdeletion of paternal origin in a 15-year-old boy with mental retardation, developmental delay, autism and congenital heart defects. Taiwanese Journal of Obstetrics & Gynecology. 2021;**60**(2):341-344. DOI: 10.1016/j.tjog.2021.01.013

[35] Azmerin M, Hussain MS, Aziz MA, Barek MA, Begum M, Sen N, et al. *TF* and *TCF4* gene polymorphisms are linked to autism spectrum disorder: A case-control study. The Journal of International Medical Research. 2022;**50**(11):3000605221138492. DOI: 10.1177/03000605221138492

[36] Battaglia A, Carey JC, South ST. Wolf-Hirschhorn syndrome: A review and update. American Journal of Medical Genetics. Part C, Seminars in Medical Genetics. 2015;**169**:216-223

[37] Fisch GS, Battaglia A, Parrini B, Youngblom J, Simensen R. Cognitive-behavioral features of children with Wolf-Hirschhorn syndrome: Preliminary report of 12 cases. American Journal of Medical Genetics. Part C, Seminars in Medical Genetics. 2008;**148C**(4):252-256. DOI: 10.1002/ajmg.c.30185

[38] Tabet AC, Verloes A, Pilorge M, Delaby E, Delorme R, Nygren G, et al. Complex nature of apparently balanced chromosomal rearrangements in patients with autism spectrum disorder. Molecular Autism. 2015;**6**:19. DOI: 10.1186/s13229-015-0015-2

[39] Morris CA. Williams syndrome. In: Adam MP, Feldman J, Mirzaa GM, et al., editors. GeneReviews®. Seattle (WA):

University of Washington; 1999, Seattle; 1993-2025

[40] Klein-Tasman BP, van der Fluit F, Mervis CB. Autism spectrum symptomatology in children with Williams syndrome who have phrase speech or fluent language. Journal of Autism and Developmental Disorders. 2018;**48**:3037-3050

[41] Driscoll DJ, Miller JL, Cassidy SB. Prader-Willi Syndrome. In: Adam MP, Feldman J, Mirzaa GM, et al., editors. GeneReviews®. Seattle (WA): University of Washington, Seattle; 1998; 1993-2025. Available from: https://www.ncbi.nlm.nih.gov/books/NBK1330/

[42] Dykens EM. Aging in rare intellectual disability syndromes. Developmental Disabilities Research Reviews. 2013;**18**:75-83

[43] Bennett JA, Germani T, Haqq AM, Zwaigenbaum L. Autism spectrum disorder in Prader-Willi syndrome: A systematic review. American Journal of Medical Genetics. Part A. 2015;**167A**(12):2936-2944. DOI: 10.1002/ajmg.a.37286

[44] AIMathews J, Williams CA. Angelman Syndrome. In: Adam MP, Feldman J, Mirzaa GM, et al., editors. GeneReviews®. Seattle (WA): University of Washington, Seattle; 1998; 1993-2025

[45] Yang L, Shu X, Mao S, Wang Y, Du X, Zou C. Genotype-phenotype correlations in Angelman syndrome. Genes (Basel). 2021;**12**(7):987. DOI: 10.3390/genes12070987

[46] Moss J, Howlin P. Autism spectrum disorders in genetic syndromes: Implications for diagnosis, intervention and understanding the wider autism spectrum disorder population. Journal of Intellectual Disability Research. 2009;**53**(10):852-873. DOI: 10.1111/j.1365-2788.2009.01197.x

[47] Lucarelli P et al. Association study of autistic disorder and chromosome 16p. American Journal of Medical Genetics. Part A. 2003;**119a**(2):242-246

[48] Taylor CM, Smith R, Lehman C, et al. 16p11.2 recurrent deletion. In: Adam MP, Feldman J, Mirzaa GM, et al., editors. GeneReviews®. Seattle (WA): University of Washington, Seattle; 2009; 1993-2025

[49] Girirajan S, Pizzo L, Moeschler J, et al. 16p12.2 recurrent deletion. In: Adam MP, Feldman J, Mirzaa GM, et al., editors. GeneReviews®. Seattle (WA): University of Washington, Seattle; 2015; 1993-2025

[50] Pizzo L, Jensen M, Polyak A, Rosenfeld JA, Mannik K, Krishnan A, et al. Rare variants in the genetic background modulate cognitive and developmental phenotypes in individuals carrying disease-associated variants. Genetics in Medicine. 2019;**21**:816-825

[51] Palumbi R, Ponzi E, Micella S, Pascali M, Bucci R, Gentile M, et al. Clinical phenotype of the 16p.13.11 microdeletion: A case report with a mini review of the literature. Frontiers in Genetics. 2024;**15**:1429185. DOI: 10.3389/fgene.2024.1429185

[52] Smith ACM, Boyd KE, Brennan C, et al. Smith-Magenis syndrome. In: Adam MP, Feldman J, Mirzaa GM, et al., editors. GeneReviews®. Seattle (WA): University of Washington, Seattle; 2001; 1993-2025

[53] Korteling D, Musch JLI, Zinkstok JR, Boot E. Psychiatric and neurological manifestations in adults with Smith-Magenis syndrome: A scoping review. American Journal of Medical Genetics.

Part B, Neuropsychiatric Genetics. 2024;**195**(2):e32956. DOI: 10.1002/ajmg.b.32956. Epub 2023 Aug 16

[54] McDonald-McGinn DM, Hain HS, Emanuel BS, et al. 22q11.2 Deletion Syndrome. In: Adam MP, Feldman J, Mirzaa GM, et al., editors. GeneReviews®. Seattle (WA): University of Washington, Seattle; 1999; 1993-2025

[55] Phelan K, Rogers RC, Boccuto L. Phelan-McDermid Syndrome-SHANK3 related. In: Adam MP, Feldman J, Mirzaa GM, et al., editors. GeneReviews®. Seattle (WA): University of Washington, Seattle; 2005; 1993-2025

[56] Asta L, Ricciardello A, Cucinotta F, Turriziani L, Boncoddo M, Bellomo F, et al. Clinical, developmental and serotonemia phenotyping of a sample of 70 Italian patients with Phelan-McDermid Syndrome. Journal of Neurodevelopmental Disorders. 2024;**16**(1):57. DOI: 10.1186/s11689-024-09572-7

[57] Soorya L, Kolevzon A, Zweifach J, Lim T, Dobry Y, Schwartz L, et al. Prospective investigation of autism and genotype-phenotype correlations in 22q13 deletion syndrome and SHANK3 deficiency. Molecular Autism. 2013;**4**(1):18

[58] Bilgeç N, Balasar Ö, Uzun N, Pekcan S, Bedel FM, Çaksen H. Case of twin achondroplasia and autism coexistence and literature review. Psychiatric Genetics. 2023;**33**(6):243-250

# Section 2

# Psychosocial Dynamics, Intervention Strategies, and Conceptual Perspectives in ASD

Chapter 4

# Fathers' and Mothers' Feedback after ASD-Modified Interaction Therapy with Their Preschool Child

*Nitza Weinstein*

## Abstract

This chapter presents qualitative research exploring the meaningful themes raised by parents following their participation in autism spectrum disorder (ASD)-Modified Interaction Therapy (IT) with their preschool-age child while comparing fathers and mothers. This 4-month, parent-mediated, interaction-focused intervention incorporates unique elements like video-based self-observation, nonjudgmental self-reflection, equal two-parent involvement, self-determined goals for change, and nonhierarchical therapist-parent collaboration. While prior research demonstrated the IT's effectiveness in enhancing parental responsiveness, affect, and attachment to their child, this study aimed to amplify parents' voices by analyzing fathers' and mothers' written feedback about their therapy's challenges and benefits. A thematic analysis of written reflections from 34 parents (20 mothers and 14 fathers) identified nine recurring themes. Parents highlighted the benefits of therapy, including increased self-awareness, more enjoyable and productive play interactions, strengthened attachment, and enhanced parenting competence. Video feedback was particularly impactful, fostering self-reflection and modifications in parents' communication patterns to meet their child's needs and communicative abilities. Parents also reported challenges like initial discomfort with videorecording, time constraints, and difficulty integrating therapeutic strategies into daily life. Notably, fathers and mothers shared similar experiences, but fathers uniquely emphasized therapists' supportive role and learning from their spouse, while mothers more frequently described affective and attachment-related benefits. Parents' feedback suggests that ASD-modified IT promotes parental empowerment and strengthens parent-child interactions. The nonhierarchical, collaborative approach supports both parents equally, encouraging individual goal-setting and mutual learning. These insights contribute to refining parent-focused interventions, emphasizing structured therapeutic spaces' facilitation of parental engagement and self-efficacy for parenting young children with ASD.

**Keywords:** brief ASD-modified interaction therapy, qualitative thematic analysis, subjective parenting experiences, therapist-parent collaboration, self-reflection, responsiveness, affect, attachment

## 1. Introduction

This chapter presents qualitative research exploring the meaningful themes raised by fathers and mothers who participated in short-term two-parent therapy with their preschool-age child with autism spectrum disorder (ASD). This 4-month multimodal parent-mediated intervention—*ASD-modified interaction therapy* (IT)—includes several unique features such as: equal participation by both parents; live parent-child interactions during free play; parents' self-reflection while investigating videotapes of their own "here and now" contribution to dyadic interaction with their child; each parent's observation of and learning from the spouse; and co-therapists' nonhierarchical, nonjudgmental collaboration with parents. Recent research demonstrated the ASD-modified IT's effectiveness for a range of ASD severity levels [1]. Expert judges rated significant improvement following therapy in both parents' responsive and affective interaction behaviors with their child, where mothers showed larger increases in affect. Mothers' self-reports also indicated the significant impact of ASD-modified IT on their pleasure during interaction and their attachment quality.

This chapter presents complementary research exploring parents' own voices related to their challenges and benefits during ASD-modified IT, which may be experienced differently by fathers and mothers. By examining parents' qualitative feedback about their therapeutic experiences and identifying patterns *via* thematic data analysis, this study aimed to deepen understanding about the IT's efficacy to promote its future refinement for both parents. Before presenting the study's findings, this introduction next reviews parents' interaction dynamics with their child with ASD, prior parent-mediated interventions targeting families, the currently investigated ASD-modified IT framework, the importance of both fathers' and mothers' involvement in therapy, and in-depth qualitative assessment evaluating parent-focused interventions.

### 1.1 Parents' interaction dynamics with a child with communication disorders

Parents of a child with ASD tend to experience complex difficulties in interacting with their child during everyday life and in establishing a close reciprocal relationship—often accompanied by parents' negative feelings like frustration, stress, resentment, and a sense of inadequacy [2]. Prior research showed the importance of parental warmth, sensitivity, responsiveness, supportive discipline, and attention-focusing to promote the child's active participation and cooperation during parent-child dyadic interactions [3]. Yet, socio-communicative deficits associated with this neurodevelopmental disorder, like children's difficulty in communicating their intentions, initiating social play, or mentalizing about others' thoughts and emotions, may also lower the likelihood of experiencing pleasant, fruitful play exchanges between parent and child [4]. In response to their child's communicative behaviors, these parents may exhibit overly controlling interaction patterns like stepping in to act on behalf of their child instead of attuning to the child and waiting to respond to the child's initiative; conversely, some parents may step away, choosing withdrawal or avoidance [5]. In turn, children with ASD who experience such parental behavior patterns may tend to increase their avoidant and repetitive behavior, which can make the interaction even more challenging for parents [6, 7].

### 1.2 Parent-mediated interventions targeting families of a child with ASD

Given that parents are the principal agents of change in the various spheres of the child's life—those who form the child's initial experiences of social interaction—parent-mediated interventions are a highly recommended modality for families of a child with ASD, to help parents learn to match their communication and play levels with their child's abilities and to engage their child in productive and enjoyable joint play interactions [8]. Evidence has suggested the efficacy of interventions for children with ASD where caregivers are actively taught to respond, play, and synchronize with their child's attentional focus [9–12]. When parents play the role of mediating agent or co-facilitator in interaction-based therapy, they can actively practice new behavior techniques with their child [13, 14].

Beyond effects on parenting skills and child variables, research studies indicated that early interventions for parents of children with ASD offer numerous psychosocial parenting-related benefits, including increases in parental empowerment and parenting self-efficacy levels. Parents who participated in treatment programs for their child with ASD, especially with video feedback, reported a higher sense of competence than untreated parents [11, 13, 14]. McConachie and Diggle [15] suggested that hands-on parent-mediated treatments are particularly beneficial to help parents understand skills and strategies for younger children. Hohlfeld et al.'s [16] systematic review of programs that directly trained parents of children with various disabilities, including ASD, revealed especially robust outcomes for enhancing parenting self-efficacy levels in parents of young children under age 5.

### 1.3 The ASD-modified IT framework

The qualitative research study presented in this chapter examines a unique parent-mediated intervention: the ASD-modified IT, a 4-month multimodal two-parent intervention aiming to promote father-child and mother-child interactions with their preschool-age child with ASD. This short-term therapy comprises Weinstein and Racheli's [4] modification of Rustin et al.'s [17] two-parent "interaction therapy" that addressed stammering to fit families of preschoolers with ASD. The ASD-modified preschooler IT was designed to help parents identify their own communication patterns through video feedback within the context of free play because of its importance in promoting reciprocal parent-child relationships [18]. Many parents do not cultivate a habit of playing with their child with ASD. The IT approach opens a doorway to play, offering both parents and the child opportunities for connection and growth. Self-awareness gained through video analysis and autonomous goal-directed play practice allows parents to better understand their young child's interaction patterns and to adapt their own communication patterns to meet their child's specific needs, aiming to enhance their quality of interaction and the child's pragmatic communicative ability. For this therapy's structure and session contents, see **Table 1**.

| Structure | Contents |
|---|---|
| Session 1:<br>• Contract (without child) | • Coordination of expectations<br>• Therapy contract: Both parents commit to participating in all sessions |
| Sessions 2–8:<br>• Core sessions of parent-child free-play interaction<br>• Each session follows a structured 4-stage process | **Stage A. Video recording**:<br>• Each parent is recorded separately during 5–7-minute free-play interaction with their child<br>• Co-therapists do not intervene |
| | **Stage B. Video viewing with co-therapists:**<br>• Before viewing the video, parents are instructed to identify:<br>1. One aspect of their behavior they believe positively contributes to verbal or nonverbal communication with their child<br>2. One behavior they would like to change |
| | **Stage C. Video analysis and selection of targeted change tasks:**<br>• Co-therapists hold dialogs with each parent to help them analyze their videotaped interaction<br>• The non-analyzing parent does not interfere while practicing listening and observing skills<br>• Parents are first invited to share a positive videotaped behavior (e.g., "I sat where my child could make eye contact")<br>• And then one behavior they want to change (e.g., "I talked too much and did not follow my child's play enough")<br>• Co-therapists help each parent understand how modifying this behavior could address their child's pragmatic communication challenges (e.g., "Yes, when you talk 'too much,' as you say, your child may feel overwhelmed. This might make your child pull away or become more passive") |
| | **Stage D. Formulation of homework assignment:**<br>• Co-therapists help each parent develop and formulate realistic, achievable homework tasks that align with their personality and parenting style<br>• For example, if "talking too much" is the parent's chosen target for improvement: "During playtime, I will focus on reducing my verbal input and creating opportunities for shared attention and/or action with my child"<br>• Together, they brainstorm strategies the parent can use during "special time" at home to apply chosen task |
| • Each parent separately practices the chosen task at home | **At-home "Special Time" (between sessions):**<br>• Special time is free-play father-child and mother-child dyadic time lasting at least 5–7 minutes, 4–6 times weekly<br>• Each parent separately practices the chosen task for change and reports their experiences in writing |
| **Session 9:** Summary meeting (without child) | • Parents each bring written feedback reflecting the process they underwent, noting positive aspects and challenges/difficulties<br>• Session concludes with a discussion on how to sustain changes in interaction patterns |

**Table 1.**
*ASD-modified interaction therapy structure and contents.*

The ASD-modified IT method derives from intersubjectivity theory and includes several major principles (see [1]): (1) equal, nonhierarchical, reciprocal partnership between the two co-therapists and each parent. Therapists and parents collaboratively construct knowledge and define goals through dynamic, circular, and productive dialog, negotiation, and interaction [19, 20]. (2) Each parent's nonjudgmental self-observation and self-reflection on their videotaped dyadic free-play interactions with their child, to raise awareness about parents' own "here-and-now" contribution. (3) Equal, uninterrupted participation by both parents to foster mutual listening and learning while empowering each parent's sense of worth and providing therapeutic space for the less-heard parent, potentially shifting family dynamics and roles. (4) Self-determined goals for therapy by each parent to highlight parents' personal responsibility and restore their sense of control and competence.

Although positive clinical impressions for ASD-modified IT have accumulated over the years, the method's efficacy was only empirically demonstrated recently. Weinstein and Zloof Golombick [1] examined the effects of manualized ASD-modified IT for 21 father-child and 21 mother-child dyads with a preschool-age child with ASD (17 boys and 4 girls) while comparing fathers and mothers. Pretest and posttest data included: expert judges' analysis of videotaped father-child and mother-child interactions to assess parental responsiveness and affect; and parent questionnaires on perceived attachment to the child. Despite the brief duration of the therapy, expert judges' ratings of parents' *in vivo* interactive behavior demonstrated rapid significant improvement in both fathers' and mothers' responsiveness and affect toward the child. Mothers' increased affect was stronger than fathers', and only mothers also showed two areas of significant improvement in their perceived attachment indices regarding their experience of pleasure during parent-child interaction and their quality of attachment to their child (see Weinstein and Zloof Golombick [1] for more details). The present qualitative study complements the prior research to further elucidate parents' voices related to the benefits and challenges of ASD-modified IT and to explore fathers' versus mothers' therapeutic experiences related to parenting a child with ASD.

### 1.4 Involving both fathers and mothers in therapy

The ASD-modified IT's distinct structured approach—enabling each parent's own equal space and time to play with their child, analyze videotapes, and formulate their own self-determined therapy goals—addresses the need to account for possible differences in fathers' versus mothers' parenting styles [21, 22] and play/language patterns with their child [23–25]. During play, compared to mothers, fathers may engage in more active rough-and-tumble play and more elaborated play that stretches beyond toys' physical properties and involves enjoyment and inventiveness [26, 27]. Such play can be very helpful and motivating for children with ASD. Optimally, therapeutic intervention should focus on each parent's strengths and parenting styles to promote their child's development and their own rewarding interactions with the child [27].

### 1.5 In-depth qualitative assessment to evaluate parent-focused interventions

Some prior researchers have conducted qualitative studies examining parent-mediated interventions. In a study comparing mothers' and fathers' evaluations about the acceptability of parent-child interaction therapy (PCIT), mothers rated PCIT significantly higher than fathers [28]. In Woodfield and Cartwright's [29] qualitative research examining feedback on the PCIT, parents initially felt self-conscious, awkward, and inadequate in utilizing new parenting skills and tools but gradually felt more natural, confident, and optimistic following repeated practice. Parents underscored the surprising effectiveness of child-led play in the PCIT and highlighted their coach's central role in promoting change. Im-Bolter and de la Roche's [30] qualitative study on parents who implemented the TalkAbility™ social-communication intervention also described growth in their own confidence, knowledge, patience, sense of empowerment, and even their mindset regarding their child's autism diagnosis and their own skills for implementing naturalistic strategies with their child. Parents accentuated the effectiveness of the flexible TalkAbility™ structured and unstructured play strategies, which could be applied to meet their child's needs in different daily contexts.

## 2. Method

### 2.1 Participants

Participants were 34 parents (20 mothers and 14 fathers) from 19 families (including one same-sex couple) who (a) completed two-parent ASD-modified IT in 2022–2024 within special-education ASD preschools that their children attended and (b) submitted feedback in the summary session. **Table 2** presents sample characteristics. Four husbands who participated fully in treatment but did not submit feedback were excluded from the study. It is worth noting that the two mothers in Family 13 participated equally in two-parent therapy, and both were analyzed as mothers.

| Family no. | Participating parents | | Child demographics | | |
|---|---|---|---|---|---|
| | Fathers ($n$ = 14) | Mothers ($n$ = 20) | Functioning level | Age (years)[a] | Sex |
| 1 | | X | Low | 3.5 | F |
| 2 | X | X | Low | 5.0 | M |
| 3 | X | X | Medium | 4.9 | M |
| 4 | | X | Medium | 4.9 | M |
| 5 | X | X | Medium | 4.9 | M |
| 6 | X | X | Low | 5.0 | M |
| 7 | X | X | Low | 5.1 | M |
| 8 | X | X | Medium | 5.0 | M |
| 9 | X | X | Low | 6.0 | M |
| 10 | X | X | Medium | 5.0 | M |
| 11 | X | X | High | 4.5 | M |
| 12 | X | X | High | 4.5 | M |
| 13 | | XX[b] | Low | 3.5 | M |
| 14 | X | X | Low | 3.8 | M |
| 15 | | X | Medium | 5.6 | M |
| 16 | X | X | High | 5.0 | F |
| 17 | X | X | High | 4.5 | M |
| 18 | | X | Medium | 3.1 | M |
| 19 | X | X | Medium | 5.5 | M |

[a]*Age at start of intervention.*
[b]*Same-sex couple.*

**Table 2.**
*Parent and child characteristics.*

Each family's preschool-age child (2 girls and 17 boys) had received an ASD diagnosis per *DSM-5* criteria [31] by a child development institute. Mothers were ages 29–41 and had 13.6 years of education on average at the start of families' participation in treatment; fathers were ages 33–49 years and had 13.0 years of education on average; preschoolers with ASD were ages 3–6 years ($M$ = 4.7) and varied in functioning level: 7 with low functioning, 8 with medium functioning, and 4 with high functioning.

### 2.2 The ASD-modified IT procedure and co-therapists

Two professional co-therapists who were multidisciplinary therapeutic staff members in the special-education ASD preschools were assigned to each family participating in the ASD-modified IT [4]. Sessions were held every other week over 3–4 months, with access to indoor toys and games, totaling 9 one-hour sessions. See **Table 1** for sessions' structure and contents. In each co-therapist pair, at least one was always a speech therapist to address core ASD communication deficits, and the other was a clinical, developmental, occupational, or art therapist. All therapists had specialized ASD expertise and at least 2 years of experience working with children and parents in the preschool setting. All therapists were supervised by the author once every 2 weeks throughout the whole process of therapy.

### 2.3 Study measure

To explore the subjective meaning that parents ascribed to their experiences during the ASD-modified IT, they received a general homework assignment near the end of treatment asking them to give written "feedback" about "what benefited or contributed to them" and "what challenges they experienced" during the 4-month intervention. No other instructions were given. Parents submitted their written feedback in their final summarizing session. The verbatim excerpts cited below underwent back-and-forth translation to English by native Hebrew and English speakers and have been anonymized to protect the families' confidentiality.

#### *2.3.1 Thematic analysis*

Qualitative methodologies adopt an inductive or "bottom-up" approach to collate parents' experiences and generate new knowledge and understanding. In this study, parents' feedback was analyzed according to Braun and Clarke's [32] six-phase model for thematic analysis. First, all of the parents' written utterances were read, taking notes of ideas and keywords that fit the general guidelines parents had received for preparing their feedback: what benefited or contributed to parents and what challenges parents experienced during the ASD-modified IT. After identifying relevant utterances, they were assembled into two categories: benefits and challenges. Next, data were re-examined for utterances related to recurring themes repeated in parents' feedback, although no clues had been provided to them about these specific themes. Repeated specific patterns were noted that appeared to be highly relevant and significant for understanding the meaning of the therapy for parents while separating fathers from mothers. Then, common concepts were combined to create themes, where each theme contained parents' detailed utterances verbatim to form deep, rich observations on the meaning that parents attributed to therapy.

## 3. Results and discussion

Overall, nine themes were identified in the parents' feedback data. Beyond the general themes of "benefits of therapy" (Theme 1) and "challenges faced in therapy" (Theme 2) that were elicited directly, seven additional recurring themes emerged from the thematic analysis of parents' verbatim transcripts, as follows: (1) therapy benefits in general; (2) therapy's challenges in general; (3) video-focused analysis and self-reflection; (4) formulation of specific targets for parent-child interaction; (5) observing and learning from spouse; (6) therapists' contribution; (7) play abilities and pleasure from interaction; (8) attachment and closeness to child; and (9) sense of competence and self-efficacy.

**Table 3** maps which of the 34 mothers and fathers mentioned each of the nine themes in their feedback concerning their experiences participating in ASD-modified IT, as well as the total number of parents who raised each theme in their feedback. **Table 4** presents some verbatim excerpts related to each theme. The discussion of these qualitative findings below includes an examination of how these themes support the main principles of ASD-modified IT (see Section 1.3 above) and the contribution of particular feedback themes to further improve the therapeutic process.

### 3.1 Theme 1: Therapy benefits in general

Thematic analysis identified 16 parents—8 of the 14 fathers (57.1%) and 8 of the 20 mothers (40.0%)—comprising almost half (47%) of the participants overall, who generally referred to the benefits of participating in ASD-modified IT (see **Table 3**). As seen in the sample excerpts presented in **Table 4**, these parents expressed the unexpected, meaningful, exciting, insightful, and successful therapeutic processes that improved their lives. Their descriptions of therapeutic benefits support other qualitative studies of parents' experiences with different interventions like PCIT [29] and TalkAbility™ [30]. For example, several parents (Fathers 5, 9; Mother 11) emphasized the benefit of being able to transfer the insights that they gained via the treatment process to other relationship systems in daily life, like their spouse and friends, in line with Jurek et al.'s [33] assertion that support skills and strategies taught within parent-implemented programs can be generalized across numerous contexts. A few parents specified the great feeling associated with their regular participation in the therapy within the preschool settings, which enabled them to feel more involved in therapy and also to become better acquainted with the nature of their child's treatments in the preschool generally (see Father 8; Mothers 1, 18).

### 3.2 Theme 2: Therapy's challenges in general

Thematic analysis identified 10 parents—5 of the 14 fathers (35.7%) and 5 of the 20 mothers (25%)—comprising 29.4% of the participants overall, who referred generally to the challenges posed by the ASD-modified IT's setting and demands. For example, some parents (e.g., Mothers 10, 15; Father 5) described their difficulty with the brief strict time allocated to each parent-child interaction in each session, which sometimes did not allow them "to adjust and feel natural" (Father 5) or did not give them enough time to play with their child: "Because the amount of time for playing was very short, I sometimes felt like I was forcing him to play, and it felt uncomfortable" (Mother 10).

| Family | Parent | General benefits | General challenges | Video/ reflection | Specific targets | Spouse learning | Therapist contribution | Play/ pleasure | Attachment | Competence |
|---|---|---|---|---|---|---|---|---|---|---|
| 1 | Mother | ✓ | ✓ | ✓ | ✓ | | | ✓ | ✓ | |
| 2 | Father | | | | ✓ | | | | | |
| | Mother | | | | ✓ | | | ✓ | | |
| 3 | Father | | ✓ | ✓ | ✓ | | | | | |
| | Mother | | ✓ | ✓ | ✓ | | | | | |
| 4 | Mother | | | ✓ | ✓ | | | | | |
| 5 | Father | ✓ | ✓ | ✓ | ✓ | ✓ | ✓ | | ✓ | |
| | Mother | | | | ✓ | | | | | |
| 6 | Father | ✓ | ✓ | ✓ | ✓ | ✓ | ✓ | ✓ | | |
| | Mother | | | ✓ | ✓ | ✓ | | ✓ | | |
| 7 | Father | | | ✓ | ✓ | | | | | |
| | Mother | | | ✓ | ✓ | | | | | |
| 8 | Father | ✓ | | ✓ | ✓ | | ✓ | ✓ | | ✓ |
| | Mother | ✓ | | | ✓ | | | | ✓ | ✓ |
| 9 | Father | ✓ | ✓ | | ✓ | ✓ | | | ✓ | |
| | Mother | ✓ | | ✓ | | | | ✓ | ✓ | |
| 10 | Father | | | | | | | | | |
| | Mother | | ✓ | | | | | | | ✓ |
| 11 | Father | | | | ✓ | | | ✓ | | |
| | Mother | ✓ | | ✓ | ✓ | | | | | |
| 12 | Father | | | | ✓ | | | | | ✓ |
| | Mother | | | | ✓ | | | | | ✓ |

| Family | Parent | General benefits | General challenges | Video/ reflection | Specific targets | Spouse learning | Therapist contribution | Play/ pleasure | Attachment | Competence |
|---|---|---|---|---|---|---|---|---|---|---|
| 13 | Mother A | ✓ | | ✓ | ✓ | | | | | |
| | Mother B | | ✓ | ✓ | ✓ | | | | | |
| 14 | Father | ✓ | | ✓ | | | ✓ | | | ✓ |
| | Mother | ✓ | | | ✓ | | | | | ✓ |
| 15 | Mother | | ✓ | | ✓ | | | ✓ | ✓ | |
| 16 | Father | ✓ | | ✓ | ✓ | | | ✓ | | ✓ |
| | Mother | ✓ | | ✓ | ✓ | | | ✓ | | ✓ |
| 17 | Father | ✓ | | | | | | ✓ | | |
| | Mother | | | | | | | ✓ | ✓ | |
| 18 | Mother | ✓ | ✓ | ✓ | ✓ | | | ✓ | | |
| 19 | Father | ✓ | | | | | | | | |
| | Mother | | | ✓ | ✓ | | | ✓ | | |
| Fathers' total *n* | | 8 | 5 | 7 | 10 | 3 | 4 | 5 | 2 | 4 |
| Mothers' total *n* | | 8 | 5 | 12 | 17 | 1 | 0 | 9 | 5 | 5 |
| Parents' total *n* | | 16 | 10 | 19 | 27 | 4 | 4 | 14 | 7 | 9 |
| (%) | | –47% | –26.50% | –55.90% | –79.40% | –11.70% | –11.70% | –41.20% | –20.60% | –26.50% |

**Table 3.**
*Thematic analysis of fathers' (n = 14) and mothers' (n = 20) feedback on ASD-modified interaction therapy.*

| Theme | Fathers | Mothers |
|---|---|---|
| 1. Therapy benefits in general | • *I use many of the insights gained through this therapy in many other relationships and life interactions. (5)*<br>• *I feel that E. and both us parents benefited equally... (6)*<br>• *Our entering the preschool regularly strengthened E.'s sense of home in this setting and enabled us to feel involved... and get to know his treatments generally. (8)*<br>• *Before therapy I was quite skeptical, even against it, feeling somehow that N. had reached his glass ceiling... But from the first meeting I saw how that glass ceiling breaks. (9)*<br>• *Improvement... can happen in such a short time. (19)* | • *I was surprised by how precisely and easily my behavior patterns changed. How the smallest things... became so clear and how those small changes brought amazing results. (1)*<br>• *Knowing that I have "homework" and will have to report on it during the next session helped me cope with my personally holding back when I felt rejected or he lacked interest. (8)*<br>• *Therapy... helped me be more realistic and lower my expectations about how things should have been. (11)*<br>• *It was very exciting to see session-to-session changes and progress in his communication and verbal abilities. Even his ability to separate from me. (14)*<br>• *I'm glad therapy brought us inside the preschool and enabled cross-fertilization. (18)* |
| 2. Therapy's challenges in general | • *Fear that he will not cooperate and frustration from transitions in the therapy setting. (3)*<br>• *I lacked time with Y. during interaction in the therapy room which sometimes did not allow me to adjust and feel natural. (5)*<br>• *Only in the middle did I stop being stressed and nervous before meetings, thinking I'm going to play in front of the camera. (6)*<br>• *Focusing on home training wasn't easy with... our tight schedules. (9)* | • *Watching video was quite challenging. (1)*<br>• *His transition from therapy room to preschool was very challenging. (3)*<br>• *At first I was stressed by... playing with him several times weekly... I did not think I could commit to it and report it. (10)*<br>• *Personally, I did not like to watch myself on video. (13B)*<br>• *I needed more time for playing during sessions.... It wasn't simple to implement playtime at home with... our schedules. (15)* |
| 3. Video-focused analysis and self-reflection | • *Without video, it would have been a post-analysis that I think contributes less than watching the interaction itself. (5)*<br>• *Generally [video] is powerful... you can follow yourself playing and identify components and interactions (some of which are complex and hard to identify), which later became key points for me. (6)*<br>• *Self-reflection and in vivo experiencing were very different from theoretical knowledge and really contributed to changes I made in my behavior. (8)*<br>• *I was glad to gain another perspective that facilitated my communication and play with E... to better understand how he sees me. (10)* | • *Watching video I really enjoyed L.'s responses and learned from them. (1)*<br>• *It was interesting to observe and analyze my and I.'s play... Strengths emerged and issues to improve in communicating and playing. (4)*<br>• *By watching E.'s responses to my behavior, I learned what I should change. (6)*<br>• *It was surprising to observe A.'s enjoyment watching our videos... with us... It helped me see points that I did not feel while playing live and to watch developments and changes in those points. (7)*<br>• *The process helped me to observe myself from outside first with the video-camera and then also at home without the camera. (11)*<br>• *I understood better what reciprocity is and what I should do to improve it. (13A)*<br>• *Analysis and self-reflection helped me understand how to approach M. in different situations. (13B)*<br>• *I learned... ways for me to... give him time and space to express himself. (14)*<br>• *I took from the process mainly... what worked and what did not work... and how to generalize it to other situations. (18)*<br>• *I learned... how I can interpret S.'s responses to play differently. (19)* |

| Theme | Fathers | Mothers |
|---|---|---|
| 4. Formula-tion of specific targets for parent-child interaction | • *Experiencing home training focused on a specific target helped... To join Y.'s moments of initiative and not force on him what seems right to me... to maintain physical contact, to hold him with me. (5)*<br>• *Turn-taking in simple basic play like with a ball. (6)*<br>• *To look for symmetrical interaction with E. where I can say "I want things" and challenge him to cope. (8)*<br>• *To accept moments of quiet and not fill every moment with talk... not to stick to rules but let interaction flow. (11)* | • *Every target for change was meaningful for me, was implemented, and still accompanies me. (1)*<br>• *To find strategies to attract I.'s attention and to increase his initiation and lead... using variation. (2)*<br>• *To use physical contact which helps A. focus... To slow my pace and to give him more time to respond... To look for laughter. (18)* |
| 5. Observing/ learning from spouse | • *Although my wife and I joked about who is more successful in breaking the ice with E., I didn't feel any competition. Rather, I learned to appreciate her patience and abilities playing with E. (6)* | • *Watching my husband playing with E. was another resource in learning how to reach E. (6)* |
| 6. Co-therapists' contribution | • *The therapists helped focus and frame simple targets... Although they seemed very clear theoretically, focusing on them, practicing and implementing them... improve our daily interactions. (5)*<br>• *All learning and progress happened due to the professionalism and sensitivity of the amazing team that supported us and taught us with lots of dedication. (14)* | — |
| 7. Play abilities and pleasure from interaction | • *I can play with E. and enjoy it when I put aside my high expectations based on how typically developing children should play. If E. can enjoy it, I can too.... At first, 5 minutes of playing felt like an eternity. Today I sometimes force myself to stop playing after 20 minutes. (6)* | • *Playtime became enjoyable for us both. (1)*<br>• *I went back to playing games with N. and not just cooking with him. (9)*<br>• *I discovered new play abilities in a new environment. (18)*<br>• *I now play with him alone, separately from his sister. (19)* |
| 8. Attachment and closeness to child | • *Therapy processes meaningfully contributed to my relations with Y. (5)* | • *Our relations became stronger, and I'm sure this therapy contributed. (1)*<br>• *There was a change in my relations with E. And in his compliance to me. (8)* |
| 9. Sense of competence and self-efficacy | • *I added new tools to my daily toolbox for communicating with E. (8)*<br>• *I feel more competent in playing with my child. (12)* | • *I feel more confident and competent in attracting him to a shared game. (8)*<br>• *Therapy made me feel more competent as a parent to a child with ASD. (12)* |

*Note. Parents' assigned numbers appear in parentheses (see* **Table 1**).

**Table 4.**
*Sample written feedback excerpts from fathers and mothers.*

*DOI: http://dx.doi.org/10.5772/intechopen.1009855*

Other parents noted their difficulty in committing to systematically playing with their child several times a week at home, explaining that a focus on home training was not easy with all their other activities and tight schedules (Father 9, Mother 15). They also pinpointed the challenge of reporting on those home-based play sessions in writing: "I didn't think I could commit to it and report on it" (Mother 10).

In their written feedback, some parents expressed a challenge related to their initial nervous tension about being filmed by the video camera (Father 6; Mothers 1, 13B). However, this low number of parents who wrote about the sense of feeling threatened by the camera was surprising compared to parents' level of discomfort and adverse reactions that were observable clinically during the initial period of treatment. Perhaps because the written feedback was collected in the final summarizing session, by this time, parents were probably more comfortable being filmed and even aware of the camera's positive benefits and power, possibly no longer viewing it as a challenge.

One family described their anxiety about their child's reaction to the transitions required by the therapy's setting. Both parents in Family 3 mentioned that their son struggled in returning to the preschool classroom after the videotaped child-parent interactions while his parents remained in the therapy room (Father 3, Mother 3). With time, it seemed that their child became accustomed to the therapy's setting, and the parents became more relaxed. It was interesting that more parents did not write up this concern in their feedback, given that initially, many parents had worried about how their child would cope because dealing with change and transition was a common challenge for their child with ASD.

### 3.3 Summary of themes 1 and 2 acceptability

In parents' general feedback, fathers did not seem to differ from mothers in the contents of their perceptions about therapy's benefits or in the challenges they faced, like making time to participate in the therapy itself or to complete homework tasks. These findings lend support to Bagner and Eyberg [34], who found that when fathers are encouraged and given the opportunity to participate in their child's treatment, they are as likely to attend sessions as frequently as mothers. Interestingly, more fathers than mothers pinpointed benefits in their feedback, which differed from prior research where mothers rated their parent-mediated intervention (PCIT) higher than fathers [28]. Perhaps this can be attributed to the current therapy's structured allocation of equal status and time for the father during intervention.

Next, the seven additional recurring themes will be presented (Themes 3–9), which emerged from the qualitative data (see **Tables 3** and **4**), beyond the general benefits and challenges that parents described in response to the therapists' request.

### 3.4 Theme 3: Video-focused analysis and self-reflection

Thematic analysis identified 19 parents—7/14 fathers (50%) and 12/20 mothers (60%)—comprising over half (55.9%) of the participants, who referred to the videotaping as an important tool that helped them to self-reflect and analyze their interactions with their child. Parents, especially mothers, described the video analysis tool as enabling deep, thorough self-given feedback that allowed them to gain life-changing perspectives and insights; successfully identify their child's needs; and modify their own behavior patterns in ways that improved their quality of interaction with their child. For example, Father 7 stated: "The video camera helped me to see myself from another perspective and to make more precise adaptations in my joint play with A."

Importantly, parents noted that observing their own videotapes helped them to notice issues of which they were unaware during their *in vivo* play session, enabling them "to watch changes in those issues over time" (Mother 7) and "to observe minor things that you would never notice otherwise" (Mother 3).

Importantly, some parents described their process of internalizing the experience of observing themselves from the outside, even without the presence of the video camera. For example, Mother 1 shared: "With time, I needed to watch the video less and less and already was able to understand during the play interaction itself what I have to keep doing and what I have to improve." Overall, the salience of this theme in parents' feedback supports prior research suggesting that personalized video feedback regarding parent-child interactions may be more influential and more likely to be remembered by parents than the use of general examples by therapists [30].

### 3.5 Theme 4: Formulation of specific targets for parent-child interaction

Thematic analysis identified 27 parents—10/14 fathers (71.4%) and 17/20 mothers (85%)—comprising the majority (79.4%) of participants, whose feedback referred explicitly to the targets for change that they had selected autonomously during the IT process. Mothers' stronger emphasis on their choices of specific targets for change, compared to fathers, may coincide with prior research indicating that mothers may tend to focus more on enhancing their child's long-term development [3, 35]. Parents' specific targets guided them during their play interactions with their child, both in preschool sessions and during the structured "special time" homework sessions. In their feedback, parents referred enthusiastically to the possibility of experiencing new targets to try during their active play interactions with their child, emphasizing the importance of gaining new knowledge through play experiences (Fathers 5, 9). This theme coincides with Woodfield and Cartwright's [29] findings on parents' positive experience of being coached in real time with their child in the PCIT intervention. Specific tasks that the current parents discussed in their written feedback included:

- To be more playful, use affect and physical contact, and look for shared enjoyment (Fathers 5, 7, 16, 17; Mothers 2, 6, 11, 14, 15, 16, 17, 18).

- To broaden and lengthen the play interaction using a variety of ideas (Fathers 7, 11; Mothers 14, 15, 16).

- To give the child a longer response time (while the parent waits), which increases the child's chance to initiate (Fathers 2, 3, 5, 7, 11; Mothers 2, 5, 7, 17, 18).

- To adjust position to enable eye contact (Fathers 3, 5, 7; Mothers 2, 5).

- To use fewer questions during interaction, decrease speech quantity, and find balance between silence and speech, between having fun and challenging the child (Fathers 2, 5, 11, 16; Mothers 4, 5, 6, 7, 13B, 19).

- To increase interaction reciprocity by stressing parental presence and will in the interaction (Fathers 2, 6, 8, 12, 17; Mothers 6, 7, 8, 17).

- To follow the child's lead and pace, join his/her initiations, not force what seems right to the parent or stick to rules or scenarios that the parent had in mind (Fathers 3, 5, 11, 17; Mothers 2, 3, 4, 11). This last target for change seemed to substantiate Woodfield and Cartwright's [29] qualitative findings from the PCIT intervention, indicating that the child-led principle is viewed by parents as surprisingly effective.

These self-determined targets for change, chosen with no prescribed direction from the co-therapists and no modeling of interactive behavior by therapists, were mostly connected to parents' responsiveness during interaction (e.g., try to be more sensitive to the child's interests, wait longer before reacting, try different strategies to gain the child's attention). The responsiveness parameter was analyzed in previous research and showed significant improvement from pretest to posttest in both fathers and mothers [1]. Fewer selected targets for change related to parental affect during preschool and homework play sessions. Yet, more mothers (40%) than fathers (28.6%) mentioned these affect-related targets in their feedback (e.g., playfulness, physical contact, enjoyment), which may help explain mothers' larger increase in affect that emerged from prior quantitative research in a different sample [1].

### 3.6 Theme 5: Observing and learning from spouse

Thematic analysis identified 4 parents—3/14 fathers (25.4%) and 1/20 mothers (5%)—comprising 11.7% of the participants overall, who referred to their spouse and the benefits of observing their spouse and their child's feedback to their spouse. For example, Father 5 explained: "Observing my wife's interaction with Y. contributed and made me think how I would act in this situation and what I can learn from her." Father 9 even wrote: "I watched N.'s behavior playing with my wife and how successful she was in building a quality connection with him, and I understood that his abilities are higher than I assumed." Woodfield and Cartwright [29] likewise found that parents in the PCIT intervention reported gaining awareness of their partner's strengths and skills and spoke of a calmer household where adults worked together more effectively to meet the child's needs. One father (6) hinted at the possibility of competition or comparison between spouses: "... [we] joked about who is more successful." Yet, fathers' ability to acknowledge their spouse's value was not accompanied by any hint of feelings of inferiority in comparison with mothers' supposedly more intuitive parenting skills [29]. However, perhaps mothers' paucity of acknowledgment of their spouse's value is related to mothers' sense of self-sufficiency and possibly even feelings of dominance in parenting their child.

### 3.7 Theme 6: Therapists' contribution

Thematic analysis identified 4 fathers, but no mothers, whose feedback referred to the therapists' contribution, comprising over one-fourth (28.5%) of the participating fathers—11.7% of the whole sample. Surprisingly, only fathers spoke about the co-therapists' contribution, enthusiastically stressing the therapists' meaningful and elucidating support and expressing gratitude for the therapists' important role in helping them formulate targets for homework and offering a sensitive, safe atmosphere conducive to feelings of competence. For example, Father 6 reported: "I needed therapists' support in shedding light on the complicated and hidden aspects and also on the aspects that seemed clear and obvious to me. The therapists' support was, in my opinion, meaningful in building my self-confidence and trust in the therapy process.... I think that the fact the therapy was conducted by two therapists added important and interesting aspects and points of view." Father 8 highlighted the therapist-parent nonhierarchical relations, coinciding with one of the main principles underlying ASD-modified IT: "The reciprocity in parents'–therapists' dialogue was inspiring and answered my need to be exposed to other perspectives about our parenting." He clarified that this mutual dialog could lead to his child's more holistic treatment: "I wanted to take advantage of the opportunity to share my knowledge and my point of view in relation to E. and his challenges and, by sharing our different knowledge, to sharpen the focus and improve all of E.'s therapies."

This theme coincided with qualitative reports following other parent-mediated interventions [29, 30], where parents pinpointed the importance of therapists' optimism, professionalism, enthusiasm, and coaching to help support their skill acquisition, highlight their strengths, and foster a sense of empowerment. However, those prior studies suggested that seeking professional intervention was difficult for fathers, whereas in the current intervention, fathers were the ones to vocalize their appreciation for the therapeutic setting. Perhaps because mothers are usually more involved in therapeutic interventions and are exposed more to therapists' consulting and support, they did not feel the need to explicitly acknowledge the therapists' role, whereas for fathers, the commitment to such an intervention is quite a new experience. Rankin et al. [36] reported that fathers were infrequently involved in intervention and general caregiving, although fathers demonstrated important contributions to their children with ASD. Another possible explanation may be the ASD-modified IT's unique nonhierarchical approach, where parents are not told what to do, are asked to autonomously select their own targets for change, and are not exposed to therapists' modeling of desired behavior—which may help fathers feel equal to therapists, valued for their opinions, and maintain locus of control, thereby promoting their willingness to seek the therapists' counsel and support.

### 3.8 Theme 7: Play abilities and pleasure from interaction

Thematic analysis identified 14 parents—5/14 fathers (35.7%) and 9/20 mothers (45%)—comprising 41.2% of the participants overall, who referred to the newfound discovery of their ability to play with their child and to enjoy it in daily life. "As a therapist myself, I have experienced playing with other kids. In this therapy I experienced playing with my own child and learned to enjoy it" (Mother 6). These parents (especially mothers) described their new understanding of the importance of play and its benefits to mutual enjoyment, reciprocity, and meaningful progress in their child's communication with them. Mother 10 noted that "even 10 minutes of playing can be of high quality." Describing exciting, mutual, fun experiences, several parents shared how they were now able to enjoy their child while playing, such as Mother 14: "To see L.'s enjoyment during play is such a pleasure for me. He is happy, laughing, and can express himself – so different from what it used to be." Father 8 summarized the benefits of playing: "Taking advantage of the therapy setting which commits you to playtime with your child, I learned to know that I benefit from playing with E. directly – from the play itself and our shared experience – and indirectly from taking time and resources to self reflect and analyze means and strategies for improving our communication and his development."

### 3.9 Theme 8: Attachment and closeness to child

Thematic analysis identified 7 parents—2/14 fathers (14.3%) and 5/20 mothers (25%)—comprising 20.6% of the participants overall, who reported that the therapy made them feel closer to their child and helped them develop a more meaningful bond. Parents described: "more acceptance, affect, physical contact, and the feeling that our relations became stronger" (Mother 9) and "some magic moments with N. that didn't happen before" (Father 9). Father 5 stated: "The therapy process meaningfully contributed to my relations with Y." In some cases, it seemed that permanent roles in family dynamics changed, as best described by Mother 15: "I was so glad and relieved that he wants to play with me. At home he always wanted to play just with his father, and I felt less significant to him. In the therapy I felt significant."

When raising a child with ASD, the child's difficulties in reciprocity may cause parents to feel rejected and decrease feelings of closeness [2]. Parents' attachment perceptions are important not only for parents' own feelings of closeness but also because secure attachments correlate significantly with these children's better functioning in relational and functional domains like pre-symbolic gestures, verbal communication, social problem-solving, imaginative thinking, and symbolic play [37].

### 3.10 Theme 9: Sense of competence and self-efficacy

Thematic analysis identified 9 parents—4/14 fathers (28.6%) and 5/20 mothers (25%)—comprising 26.5% of the participants overall, whose feedback referred to the empowerment that they experienced participating in the therapy, with improved feelings of competence and sense of self-efficacy in parenting a child with ASD, including changes in their role within the family system. Parents attributed these feelings to the self-knowledge they gained through experiencing play interactions *in vivo* and through finding the right strategies and tools that fit their personality and the needs of their child. Mother 10 shared: "I discovered that I as a parent can play with my child within the therapeutic approach. I felt we gained a very important tool to help E. in so many things and I am glad we did it." Father 14 described a sense of internalizing the therapist's role: "I feel I know what to do even when I am not told, and this gives me a lot of confidence in being with L." Parents also reported feelings of hope about the future and confidence that they will continue to improve even after therapy ends: "We gained the belief that L. will be able to continue in his progress and we are more competent in our parenting of him" (Mother 14). This finding supports Woodfield and Cartwright's [29] suggestion that speaking about seeing changes in their child brings parents a sense of hope, a belief that change is possible, and the confidence that parents can contribute greatly to this change. The level of commitment to intervention is essential for its success, especially in light of the expectation that parents could learn to implement the role of being the therapist themselves after completing therapy [38].

## 4. Conclusions

This qualitative study permitted an in-depth understanding of parents' views and lived experiences following the ASD-modified IT. In general, parents of young preschoolers with ASD expressed meaningful and enjoyable therapeutic processes that improved their lives, along with challenges that they overcame during the intervention. Some of the themes that emerged from the data's analysis coincided with the therapy's main principles. First, coinciding with this treatment's intersubjectivity approach, parents learned to view themselves as equal co-therapists in their own process, relying on their self-knowledge and knowledge of their child and sharing those with therapists through dynamic, reciprocal dialog aiming to find specific targets for change that could improve their parent-child interaction. The collaborative therapeutic relationship emphasized therapist-parent reciprocity, paralleling the desired parent-child reciprocity that therapy aimed to nurture.

Parents' feedback also indicated their adoption of a nonjudgmental investigative approach to self-observe and self-reflect on their videotaped interactions while using a beginner's open, questioning eyes, free of preconceptions or expectations [39, 40], to help shape new interpretations of reality [41]. Analysis of their feedback reveals that parents succeeded in shifting focus from observing their child to observing their own current interaction with their child, as captured on video, staying in the "here and now" instead of looking back at the past, identifying their own patterns of communication, and choosing targets for change that reflect more responsiveness and more affect, according to the needs and communicative abilities of their special child. Parents' feedback showed that they understood their behaviors' influence on their child's communication characteristics, succeeded in autonomously selecting therapy goals and formulating alternative behaviors, and discovered new play abilities that added enjoyment. Thus, parents felt more strongly attached to their child and experienced empowerment in their sense of competence and self-efficacy for parenting a child with ASD.

This qualitative analysis amplifying parents' voices revealed that fathers and mothers shared similar experiences, but fathers uniquely emphasized the therapists' supportive role and learning from their spouse, whereas mothers did not. Mothers more frequently described affective and attachment-related benefits. The current intervention outcomes on parents of young children, ages 4.7 years on average, support the effectiveness of parent-focused interventions for this age [15, 16]. Parents' ability to implement strategies that were specifically applicable to a child's behavior was instrumental in the perceived relevance of intervention [42], which is linked to increased improvements in child behavior [43].

### 4.1 Limitations

The study reported in this chapter had a relatively small sample size with one same-sex outlier, which precluded analysis by parents' demographics like age or education level. For example, Tiano et al. [28] found that older parents rated the PCIT and its components less favorably. Also, although prior quantitative research on this therapy showed no effect of children's ASD severity on parents' pre-post changes, the current sample size did not allow for analysis of its impact. Moreover, although this feedback task asked parents to report difficulties as well as benefits, possible social desirability response bias cannot be overlooked. Finally, caution should be taken in generalizing the present results because the current parents are those who completed the therapeutic process and did not drop out or decline to submit feedback. Even if they felt the therapy was very difficult, they were able to cope with the challenges and complete the process. Thus, conclusions cannot be drawn about other families who did not complete ASD-modified IT or the fathers who did not submit feedback at the end of their therapy experience.

## Acknowledgements

Appreciation is extended to the participating families, co-therapists, and the Israeli Autism Association (OTI) for integrating ASD-modified IT into their preschools, and special thanks to Dee B. Ankonina for her support and contribution to this study.

*DOI: http://dx.doi.org/10.5772/intechopen.1009855*

## Author details

Nitza Weinstein
The Israeli Autism Association (OTI), Tel Aviv, Israel

*Address all correspondence to: nitz.weinstein@gmail.com

## References

[1] Weinstein N, Zloof Golombick A. ASD-modified interaction therapy: Effects on fathers' and mothers' responsiveness, affect, and attachment. Journal of Early Intervention. 2025;**47**(1):107-124

[2] Slade A. Mentalizing the unmentalizable: Parenting children on the spectrum. Journal of Infant, Child, and Adolescent Psychotherapy. 2009;**8**(1):7-21

[3] Ostfeld-Etzion S, Feldman R, Hirschler-Guttenberg Y, Laor N, Golan O. Self-regulated compliance in preschoolers with autism spectrum disorder: The role of temperament and parental disciplinary style. Autism. 2016;**20**(7):868-878

[4] Weinstein N, Racheli O. Parent-child therapy in families of children with ASD. Speech, Language, and Hearing. 2003;**25**:49-62. (In Hebrew)

[5] O'Nions E, Happé F, Evers K, Boonen H, Noens I. How do parents manage irritability, challenging behaviour, non-compliance and anxiety in children with autism spectrum disorders? A meta-synthesis. Journal of Autism and Developmental Disorders. 2018;**48**(4):1272-1286

[6] Midouhas E, Yogaratnam A, Flouri E, Charman T. Psychopathology trajectories of children with autism spectrum disorder: The role of family poverty and parenting. Journal of the American Academy of Child & Adolescent Psychiatry. 2013;**52**(10):1057-1065

[7] Shawler PM, Sullivan MA. Parental stress, discipline strategies, and child behavior problem in families with young children with autism spectrum disorders. Focus on Autism and other Developmental Disabilities. 2017;**32**(2):142-151

[8] Freeman S, Kasari C. Parent-child interactions in autism: Characteristics of play. Autism. 2013;**17**(2):147-161

[9] Burrell TL, Borrego JJ. Parents' involvement in ASD treatment: What is their role? Cognitive and Behavioral Practice. 2012;**19**(3):423-432

[10] Karst JS, Van Hecke AV. Parent and family impact of autism spectrum disorders: A review and proposed model of intervention evaluation. Clinical Child and Family Psychology Review. 2012;**15**(3):247-277

[11] Poslawsky E, Naber F, Bakermans-Kranenburg M, Daalen E, Engelang H, IJzendoorn, M. Video-feedback intervention to promote positive parenting adapted to autism (VIPP-AUTI): A randomized controlled trial. Autism. 2015;**19**(5):588-603

[12] Smith T, Iadarola S. Evidence base update for autism spectrum disorder. Journal of Clinical Child & Adolescent Psychology. 2015;**44**(6):897-922

[13] Kasari C, Gulstrud A, Paparella T, Hellemann G, Berry K. Randomized comparative efficacy study of parent-mediated interventions for toddlers with autism. Journal of Consulting and Clinical Psychology. 2015;**83**(3):554-563

[14] Solomon R, Van Egeren A, Mahoney G, Huber M, Zimmerman P. PLAY project home consultation intervention program for young children with autism spectrum disorders: A randomized controlled trial. Journal of Developmental and Behavioral Pediatrics. 2014;**35**(8):475-485

[15] McConachie H, Diggle T. Parent implemented early intervention for young children with autism spectrum disorder: A systematic review. Journal of Evaluation in Clinical Practice. 2007;**131**(1):120-129

[16] Hohlfeld A, Harty M, Engel M. Parents of children with disabilities: A systematic review of parenting interventions and self-efficacy. African Journal of Disability. 2018;7:437

[17] Rustin L, Botterill W, Kelman E. Assessment and Therapy for Dysfluent Children: Family Interaction. London: Whurr; 1996

[18] Winnicott DW. Playing and Reality. London: Tavistock Publications, Routledge; 1971

[19] Houzel D. Working with parents of autistic children. In: Tsiantis J, Boethious SB, Hallerfors B, Horne A, Tischler L, editors. Work with Parents: Psychoanalytic Psychotherapy with Children and Adolescents. Karnac, London: Karnak Books; 2000. pp. 115-134

[20] Nave E, Yogev E. Toward a Dialogue with Yesterday. Tel Aviv Israel: Bavel; 2002. (In Hebrew)

[21] Hirschler-Guttenberg Y, Feldman R, Ostfeld-Etzion S, Laor N, Golan O. Self- and co-regulation of anger and fear in preschoolers with autism spectrum disorders: The role of maternal parenting style and temperament. Journal of Autism and Developmental Disorders. 2015a;**45**(9):3004-3014

[22] Hirschler-Guttenberg Y, Golan O, Ostfeld-Etzion S, Feldman R. Mothering, fathering, and the regulation of negative and positive emotions in high-functioning preschoolers with autism spectrum disorder. Journal of Child Psychology and Psychiatry and Allied Disciplines. 2015b;**56**(5):530-539

[23] Cohen D, Cassel RS, Saint-Georges C, Mahdhaoui A, Laznik MC, Apicella F, et al. Do parentese prosody and fathers' involvement in interacting facilitate social interaction in infants who later develop autism? PLoS One. 2013;**8**(5):1-10

[24] Flippin M, Watson LR. Fathers' and mothers' verbal responsiveness and the language skills of young children with autism spectrum disorder. American Journal of Speech-Language Pathology. 2015;**24**(3):400-410

[25] Robinson CA, York K, Rothenberg A, Bissell LJ. Parenting a child with Asperger's syndrome: A balancing act. Journal of Child and Family Studies. 2015;**24**(8):2310-2321

[26] Creighton G, Brussoni M, Oliffe J, Olsen L. Fathers on child's play: Urban and rural Canadian perspectives. Men and Masculinities. 2015;**18**(5):559-580

[27] Flippin M, Crais E. The need for more effective father involvement in early autism intervention: A systematic review and recommendations. Journal of Early Intervention. 2011;**33**(1):24-50

[28] Tiano JD, Grate RM, McNeil CB. Comparison of mothers' and fathers' opinions of parent–child interaction therapy. Child & Family Behavior Therapy. 2013;**35**(2):110-131

[29] Woodfield MJ, Cartwright C. Parent-child interaction therapy from the parents' perspective. Journal of Child and Family Studies. 2020;**29**:632-647

[30] Im-Bolter N, de la Roche L. What parents want: A qualitative analysis of a parent-implemented intervention

for autistic children. Autism and Developmental Language Impairments. 2023;**8**:1-14

[31] American Psychiatric Association. Diagnostic and Statistical Manual of Mental Disorders. 5th ed2013

[32] Braun V, Clarke V. Using thematic analysis in psychology. Qualitative Research in Psychology. 2006;**3**(2):77-101

[33] Jurek L, Leadbitter K, Falissard B, Colin C, Touzet S, Geoffray M. Parental experience of parent-mediated intervention for children with ASD: A systematic review and qualitative evidence synthesis. Autism. 2023;**27**(3):647-666

[34] Bagner DM, Eyberg SM. Father involvement in parent training: When does it matter? Journal of Clinical Child & Adolescent Psychology. 2003;**32**:599-605

[35] Román-Oyola R, Figueroa-Feliciano V, Torres-Martinez Y, Torres-Vélez J, Encarnación-Pizarro K, Fragoso-Pagán S, et al. Play, playfulness, and self-efficacy: Parental experiences with children on the autism spectrum. Occupational Therapy International. 2018;**33**:1-10

[36] Rankin JA, Paisley CA, Tomeny TS, Eldred SW. Fathers of youth with autism spectrum disorder: A systematic review of the impact of fathers' involvement on youth, families, and intervention. Clinical Child and Family Psychology Review. 2019;**22**(4):458-477

[37] Seskin L, Feliciano E, Tippy G, Yedlouts R, Sossin M, Yasik A. Attachment and autism: Parental attachment representations and relational behaviors in the parent–child dyad. Journal of Abnormal Child Psychology. 2010;**38**(7):949-960

[38] O'Toole C, Lyons R, Houghton C. A qualitative evidence synthesis of parental experiences and perceptions of parent–child interaction therapy for preschool children with communication difficulties. Journal of Speech, Language, and Hearing Research. 2021;**64**(8):3159-3185

[39] Elitsur E. Coming out of the well, a haiku for breakfast: A recommendation for therapists. "Nefesh:" A quarterly for psychology. Therapy and Creative Education. 2000;**2**:4-14. (In Hebrew)

[40] Mitchell SA. Relationality: From Attachment to Intersubjectivity. Hillsdale, NJ: Analytic Press; 2000

[41] Ezrati-Vinacour R, Weinstein N. A dialogue among various cultures and its manifestation in stuttering therapy. Journal of Fluency Disorders. 2011;**36**(3):174-185

[42] Russell KM, Ingersoll B. Factors related to parental therapeutic self-efficacy in a parent-mediated intervention for children with autism spectrum disorder: A mixed methods study. Autism. 2021;**25**(4):971-981

[43] Mackenzie EP, Fite PJ, Bates JE. Predicting outcome in behavioral parent training: Expected and unexpected results. Child and Family Behavior Therapy. 2004;**26**:37-53

Chapter 5

# Parent-Meditated Autism Intervention: Current Practice and Future Direction

*Waganesh A. Zeleke and Jihad Torky*

## Abstract

Parent-mediated interventions have emerged as a promising approach for the treatment of autism spectrum disorder (ASD). This chapter provides an evidence-based analysis of the nature, history, characteristics, current practices, and future directions of parent-mediated autism intervention programs. This highlights the crucial role of parents and caregivers in their children's developmental, social, and behavioral outcomes. This chapter provides an overview of various parent-mediated intervention frameworks, such as naturalistic developmental behavioral interventions (NDBIs), caregiver training models, and culturally responsive practices, along with case examples. The benefits of empowering parents as active participants in therapy are discussed, emphasizing the importance of tailoring interventions to align with family dynamics and systemic and cultural contexts. This chapter also addresses the risk and protective factors associated with parent-mediated interventions and their implications for long-term child and family outcomes. While parent-mediated interventions have shown effectiveness in improving communication skills, social interactions, and adaptive behaviors in children with ASD, challenges such as parental stress, maintaining treatment fidelity, and limited access to trained professionals are also acknowledged. Future directions in this field include leveraging technological advancements, developing personalized intervention approaches, expanding research to include long-term follow-up studies and cross-cultural adaptations, and advocating for increased support and resources for families with ASD. This chapter underscores the significance of continued research and development in parent-mediated interventions to enhance the quality of life of children with ASD and their families.

**Keywords:** parent-meditated, intervention, autism, caregiver training, evidence based intervention

## 1. Introduction

Autism Spectrum disorders are neurodevelopmental disorders that affect the social and communication conditions of individuals [1]. While there is no etiological base treatment has been established; different interventions have been created to address the associated defects of these disorders. The overall goal across all interventions for autism is to enhance skills and communication abilities, and support individuals within the spectrum to better adapt to their environments. Despite the mixed research results and challenges in studying autism treatment [2], it is essential to have an evidence-based intervention that guides both parents and professionals in choosing approaches to support individuals with ASD and address their needs. The types of interventions for individuals with autism can be (1) psychoeducation/behavioral, (2) psychopharmacological, and (3) less traditional or complementary [3].

This chapter intends to assess parent-mediated intervention (PMI), which is a commonly utilized psychoeducational and behavioral intervention in the autism field, aiming to offer an analysis grounded in evidence and a comprehensive look at the current theories shaping the advancement of parent-mediated intervention (PMI). It starts by introducing the essence and reasoning behind PMIs, while summarizing their evolution. After that discussion, the conceptual foundation of PMIs ensues, along with an evidence-based assessment of their elements and implementation strategies, as well as their cultural adaptation aspects and factors influencing their efficacy, followed by insights into future pathways for PMIs.

## 2. Parent mediated autism interventions

The realm of autism interventions lies in the concept of parent-mediated interventions, where parents are actively involved in training their children with autism spectrum disorder (ASD). This approach gained traction in circles following a debate on its merits and challenges [4]. The discourse primarily centers on whether such involvement adds pressure to parents or enhances the effectiveness of a child's intervention by empowering parents as participants in their child's learning journey and ultimately fostering stronger familial bonds through natural interactions that support the development of socialization skills, communication abilities, and behavioral competencies. Clinical practice and available research indicate that involving parents as co-therapists leads to outcomes for children, including financial benefits (e.g., increasing the duration of consistent intervention for the child) and improving the chances of transferring learned skills from school or specialist settings [5].

Involving parents in autism intervention programs is crucial for several reasons. First, parents play a role in maintaining consistent and meaningful interactions with their children to help generalize skills across different environments and ensure that the learned behaviors are consistently reinforced. Research suggests that interventions led by parents have shown an impact on enhancing interactions between parents and children, and boosting language abilities and social involvement [6, 7].

Additionally, involving parents in interventions helps enhance the availability and scalability of autism services to those in need of support in this area of healthcare provision. Numerous families encounter obstacles when attempting to access services for a variety of reasons, such as location limitations or financial strain, among other things that prevent them from seeking the help they need for their loved ones with autism. Parent-mediated interventions play a role in overcoming these obstacles by empowering parents to administer interventions with the assistance of telehealth services or remote guidance where necessary.

Parental education has been shown to have effects on the well-being of caregivers. Parents of children with ASD often face increased stress levels and feelings of being overwhelmed compared with parents of neurotypical children. PMI equips parents with strategies to effectively meet their child's needs, while reducing feelings of isolation and boosting their confidence [8].

The parent training program comprises two main categories: *parental support*, aimed at boosting parental knowledge, and *parent-mediated intervention (PMI)*, which focuses on equipping parents with effective techniques and skills to interact with their children with autism. Compared to parent support programs, in which children receive indirect benefits, PMI is thought to bring direct outcomes for both the child and the parent [9]. This chapter delves deeper into the aspects of parent training programs such as parent-mediated intervention (PMI).

PMI is primarily delivered by parents, primary caregivers, and family members to meet the developmental and therapeutic needs of children with autism spectrum disorders [10]. Based on the level and depth of parental engagement in the intervention process, PMI programs can be classified into two categories: *primary and complementary*. PMIs are considered the primary intervention approach when parents facilitate the intervention. The PMI can also serve as a complementary intervention in cases where the therapy begins with the child working with a therapist and later includes parents to help apply the techniques learned from therapy sessions to settings such as home, school, or clinics [9, 11].

In PMIs, there are usually two phases involved:

1. Training stage: During this stage of the process, clinicians take on the responsibility of educating, training, and guiding parents on the disorders present as well as various intervention techniques

2. Implementation stage: After training phase, parents are tasked with implementing intervention strategies based on the guidance and expertise provided by their trainers. In this stage, the professional's role is to act as a coach, offering guidance and monitoring of the parents' implementation of these techniques to ensure accuracy and effectiveness while providing support.

PMI can be delivered through:

a. Face-to-face consultation with professionals

b. Telehealth and online forums

c. A combination of both approaches.

The key difference between general PMIs and autism-focused PMIs is the specialized and personalized approach inherent in autism-focused PMI techniques that are grounded in evidence-based practices that focus on equipping parents with strategies to enhance their child's engagement, communication, and social interactions, and assist parents in reducing stress related to the burden of caregiving and raising a child with ASD [12, 13]. The intervention may incorporate techniques to improve joint attention, foster reciprocal play, or develop language skills foundational for broader developmental progress [5] while instructing parents on how to apply self-care and nurture their well-being.

## 3. The progression of parent-mediated autism interventions (PMAI): A historical perspective

The development of Parent-Mediated Autism Interventions (PMAI) reflects a broader shift in autism intervention approaches, transitioning from parental blame to clinician-led treatments and ultimately to more inclusive, family centered models. This evolution can be divided into six chronological phases.

### 3.1 Early theories and parents' role (1940s–1960s)

In the early history of autism research, parental involvement in interventions was often limited and parents were sometimes implicated in the etiology of the condition. Kanner [14] initially described autism as a neurodevelopmental disorder and noted a perceived emotional distance between the parents of children with autism, which subsequently contributed to the development of the "*refrigerator mother*" theory [15]. This hypothesis, largely influenced by psychoanalytic principles, posits that emotionally cold and detached parenting causes autism. Such theories were profoundly detrimental to families, frequently resulting in recommendations for the removal of children from their parents for treatment [16].

In the 1960s, experts began questioning these beliefs, leading to an understanding of autism as a neurological disorder. In his 1964 study, Rimland played a role in changing perspectives by rejecting explanations and highlighting the biological roots of autism. His research was instrumental in setting up the National Society for Autistic Children. Now known as the Autism Society of America in 1965 to help parents. This was a big change. Parents started to be seen as part of the solution rather than the problem.

### 3.2 Parents as partners in therapy (1970s)

In the 1970s, a shift in the role of parents occurred thanks to the work of psychologist Eric Schopler in developing the Treatment and Education of Autistic and Related Communication Handicapped Children (TEACCH) program at the University of North Carolina, along with his colleagues. In 1972, this initiative marked the inception of the autism service program at a level in the United States, focusing on engaging families and utilizing structured teaching methods that parents could apply within their homes effectively. Schoplers' groundbreaking work in his 1971 piece "Parents as co-therapists in the Treatment of Children" highlighted the significance of involvement in yielding positive outcomes for individuals with autism spectrum disorders early on in research. His findings challenged the notion of disconnect between professionals and parents. Advocated for a collaborative approach towards supporting children's progress [17, 18].

### 3.3 Expansion of parent-mediated approaches (1980s–1990s)

During the 1980s, research on child development and intervention strategies went through a shift towards valuing intervention and promoting natural parent-child interactions as crucial factors for a child's growth and progress. Various approaches, such as Applied Behavior Analysis (ABA), were introduced during this period, emphasizing involving parents to support their child's development rather than just playing passive roles. As time passed, research in the field provided evidence supporting the effectiveness of parent training programs in enhancing outcomes such as shared attention between parent and child and improvements in language skills and social interactions. The convergence of valuing developmental methods, alongside the rise of parent education, has resulted in the acceptance of PMIs.

In the '90s, Parent Training gained advancements through Applied Behavior Analysis (ABA), a groundbreaking development credited to O. Ivar Lovaas in 1987 [19]. The study by Lovaas highlighted that early intervention with 40 hours per week of ABA showed remarkable enhancements in IQ and adaptive skills for almost half of the participants as opposed to just 2% in the control group [19]. Consequently, a demand spike for interventions based on ABA was observed. When experts first introduced ABA therapy, its principles were detailed in The ME Book by Lovaas in 1981, to guide parents in using ABA methods at home. Subsequently many parents have been taught methods, like trial training and reinforcement strategies to carry out ABA interventions, within their homes [19, 20]. Meanwhile, researchers have also started looking into play-based approaches that focus on enhancing parent-child interactions. Robert and Lynn Koegel introduced a method known as Pivotal Response Training (PRT) in 1989 [21] to help parents enhance their children's motivation and social communication skills through reinforcement techniques. Similarly, Stanley Greenspan's DIR/Floor time approach, from 1997 advises parents to engage in play by following their child's led to promote participation and emotional bonding. Government policies show support for parent-involved strategies.

In the United States, during the 1986 Education of the Handicapped Act Amendments era and later reinforced by the Individuals with Disabilities Education Act in 1991, it was mandated that early intervention programs for children aged 0–3 should be centered around families with parents receiving training to support their children's development needs. During the 1990s, parent-training programs became more accessible and widespread across the nation. The EarlyBird initiative was introduced by the National Autistic Society, in the UK back in 1997 as one of the pioneering parent education programs designed to support parents of children [22]. Likewise, the "Hanen More Than Words" program emerged in Canada during the 1990s with an emphasis on providing parents with training geared towards enhancing communication skills [23].

### 3.4 Evidence-based research and global expansion (2000s)

In the 2000s there was a rise, in evidence-based research confirming the effectiveness of interventions involving parents in child development and communication skills improvement through reviews like those, from the Cochrane Collaboration and large scale randomized controlled trials assessing programs [1, 24, 25]. For example, in studies conducted in the 2000s by Bryson and McArthur, on Hanen and Developmental Social Pragmatic Interventions, it was demonstrated that language development is positively correlated with responsiveness as indicated [26].

### 3.5 Global expansion and diverse approaches (2010s–Present)

During the 2010s and beyond, there has been growth in parent-mediated interventions on a scale as they have tailored their approaches to fit different cultural and resource contexts around the world. As awareness of autism has grown globally during this time period, many regions have adopted parent training as a scalable method in areas where there is a shortage of specialists in autism. This era has been marked by advancements that have shaped the landscape of autism interventions worldwide. Substantial studies and extended results revealed that ongoing parent-mediated interventions have demonstrated advantages over time. For instance, the PACT study conducted by Pickles et al. In 2016 indicated a decrease, in the severity of autism, during adolescence.

In low resource environments programs, like the Parent-mediated intervention for autism spectrum disorder in South Asia (PASS) as shown by Rahman et al. [27] study have proven the effectiveness of training parents, in India and Pakistan. The Caregiver Skills Training (CST) program, by the World Health Organization (WHO), was created in partnership with Autism Speaks to offer group training sessions at no cost, focusing on communication skills improvement and behavior management techniques while also emphasizing self-care practices [28].

## 4. Theoretical foundations of parent-meditated intervention

Parent-mediated intervention (PMI) is an approach characterized by a complex system involving a child requiring support, parents functioning as primary caregivers, and dynamic relationships that develop between them. Professionals serve as coaches and trainers for parents by providing them with techniques to support their children.

A comprehensive examination of the PMI's theoretical framework is essential to understand this multifaceted dynamic. As **Table 1** illustrates, the PMI is grounded in and developed based on several underlying naturalistic developmental and behavioral theories, including social learning theory, attachment theory, ecological and family systems theory, applied behavioral analysis, cognitive attribution theory, and motivational interviewing. These theories elucidate how children learn, form attachments, and develop, as well as the factors that influence their behavior. The integration of these theories facilitates a more comprehensive approach to addressing complex

| Theory | Core idea | Application in PMI |
|---|---|---|
| Social Learning Theory (SLT) Albert Bandura (1977) | Children learn by observing and imitating others. | Parents model social behaviors (e.g., eye contact, turn-taking).<br>Use reinforcement to encourage imitation. |
| Attachment Theory John Bowlby (1969), Mary Ainsworth (1978) | Secure attachment fosters trust, emotional regulation, and learning. | Teaching parents to respond to children's emotional cues, Foster joint attention and build secure attachment. |
| Applied Behavior Analysis (ABA) B.F. Skinner (1953) | Behavior is influenced by reinforcement (positive/negative). | Using reinforcement, structured learning, and play-based interventions |
| Cognitive Attribution Theory Bernard Weiner (1985) | Perceptions of ability affect motivation and behavior. | Helping parents develop a growth mindset about their children's abilities. |
| Ecological theory Urie Bronfenbrenner (1979), Bowen (1985) | Child development is shaped by environmental influences (family, culture, etc.). | Considering family dynamics, cultural background, and resources to make interventions practical and effective. |
| Motivational Interviewing (MI) Miller & Rollnick (1991) | Intrinsic motivation enhances engagement and behavior change. | Empowering parents in goal setting and intervention planning.<br>Addressing barriers to engagement (e.g., stress and doubt).<br>Enhance commitment to implementing strategies consistently. |

**Table 1.**
*Summary of PMI theoretical framework.*

*DOI: http://dx.doi.org/10.5772/intechopen.1010294*

family dynamics and enhancing parent-child relationships across diverse contexts and populations.

### 4.1 Social learning theory (SLT): Observational learning and parental modeling

Bandura's (1977) Social Learning Theory (SLTs), which he developed back in the day, highlighted the significance of modeling and reinforcement in picking up behaviors through observation and imitation of others, in the surroundings of ones according to SLTs theory, children grasp skills and behaviors using four key processes that affect learning:

- Attention: The child must pay attention to the modeled behavior.
- Retention: The child must remember the observed behavior.
- Reproduction: The child must have the ability to reproduce the behavior.
- Motivation: The child must be motivated to perform the behavior, which is often influenced by reinforcement.

In the context of PMIs, social learning theory emphasizes the importance of teaching parents how to demonstrate communication skills and emotional regulation while interacting with their children. Many children diagnosed with autism spectrum disorder find it challenging to imitate behaviors and engage in exchanges naturally; hence, there is a need for clear modeling and positive reinforcement in their learning processes. PMIs utilize a combination of structured and naturalistic modeling, where parents demonstrate social behaviors (e.g., eye contact, taking, gestures), using guided participation to encourage imitation, provide positive reinforcement when a child successfully mimics or starts interactions, and integrate learning into routines to ensure that the skills generalize beyond therapy settings. For example, in Reciprocal Imitation Training (RIT), which is a type of PMI informed by SLT, parents participate in play activities in which they mimic their child's actions first to capture the child's interest and encourage reciprocal interactions. This helps the child learn to imitate their parents' social actions over time and aids in early social communication skill development [29, 30].

## 5. Attachment theory

Attachment Theory suggests that the connection between children and caregivers influences their emotional growth and cognitive development [31, 32]. When there is a secure attachment in place, it helps build trust and promotes regulation and social interaction skills; however, insecure attachment may result in anxiety or challenges in social situations leading to withdrawal.

In PMIs, numerous children with ASD exhibit behaviors, due to their sensitivity to sensory stimuli and challenges, in understanding social signals or communicating effectively with others. PMIs strive to integrate principles centered around building parent–child relationships and nurturing emotional ties that facilitate the child's educational progress. Some of the strategies employed in these programs are encompassed.

Effective PMI involves guiding parents to understand and respond to their child's emotions and signals in a manner that builds trust and promotes positive connections. Encouraging parents to acknowledge their child's feelings and building bonds through shared activities that promote enjoyment and interaction are essential strategies. Additionally, attachment theory plays a role in parent-led interventions by highlighting the significance of forming attachments between caregivers and infants for the child's future social-emotional growth [33]. Interventions such as using video feedback to encourage Positive Parenting and Sensitive Discipline (VIPPSD) along with Middle Childhood Attachment-based Family Therapy (MCAT) are based on attachment theory. They aim to foster parenting care and to establish attachment bonds [33].

## 6. Applied behavior analysis (ABA)

Based on Skinner's [34] operant conditioning model, Applied Behavior Analysis (ABA) is a method that relies on data and focuses on using reinforcement to encourage behavior change.

PMI programs integrate ABA principles using strategies to boost behavior through reinforcement methods and functional communication training (FCT) to substitute behaviors with more suitable forms of communication. Some of the known naturalistic developmental behavior-based PMIs, such as Pivotal Response Training (PRT) and the Early Start Denver Model (ESDM), incorporate ABA strategies into parent-guided play interactions.

## 7. Cognitive attribution theory

Weiner [35] proposed Attribution Theory, which states that individuals' interpretations of events can impact their motivation and actions. Parents who perceive their children's challenges related to autism as changeable are more inclined to continue the interventions.

The principles of attribution have been incorporated into many PMI program applications to assist parents in fostering an attitude towards their children's potential for growth and development. According to cognitive attribution theory, promoting belief, such as changing the mindset from "My child can't handle this" to "With some help and guidance. my child can make progress." Facilitate changes in child development.

## 8. Ecological and family systems theory

Developed by Urie Bronfenbrener [36], Ecological Systems Theory argues that children's development can be shaped or influenced by the environment in which they live. These environments, which Bronfenbrener classified into six different systems, include microsystems, mesosystems, ecosystems, exosystems, and macrosystems. A microsystem refers to a circle of family members and caregivers who provide support and care. In the mesosystem, there is a connection between the family and external entities, such as therapists and schools. Environmental factors indirectly affect ecosystems, such as the role of healthcare policies in exosystem dynamics. The macrosystem encompasses beliefs, social conventions, and resource availability.

Bowens' family systems theory [37] also underscores the impact of family dynamics, stress levels, and support systems on a child's development. This theory is applied within the realm of PMI through the acknowledgment of the importance of focusing on the needs of both the child and family in interventions. This strategy involves interventions to manage stress to enhance the well-being of parents, and understanding the impact of family beliefs and resources on the effectiveness of interventions is crucial for implementing practices. The PMI ensures that interventions for children consider their family and community contexts for practicality and adaptability in real-life situations.

## 9. Motivational interviews

Motivational interviewing (MI) is an approach to inspiring changes in individuals' lives and helping them reach their full potential. Motivational Interviewing (MI), developed by Miller and Rollnick [38], aims to help individuals make changes by tackling feelings, changing, and enhancing self-belief and inner drive. Most PMIs use MI techniques such as supporting parents to set goals and plan interventions effectively overcoming obstacles, participating in activities such as stress and uncertainty, and strengthening dedication to consistently apply strategies.

## 10. Core principles of parent mediated autism interventions

PMAI incorporates structured frameworks and strategies that have demonstrated efficacy in children with ASD. Research indicates that five key principles guide the development and implementation of Autism-focused PMIs. These include.

### 10.1 Naturalistic learning environments

Integrating interventions into natural environments, such as home, school, and community settings, is the primary aspect of PMI. Unlike therapies conducted in clinics that have structured and controlled settings for children's skill development, PMI allows children to learn and practice in familiar surroundings, leading to better generalization and retention of newly acquired behaviors [39]. Naturalistic developmental behavioral interventions (NDBIs) emphasize the importance of parents creating learning opportunities during regular daily routines to support this approach [40].

### 10.2 Collaborative and egalitarian partnership between trainers/coaches/counselors and parents

The relationship between professionals acting as mentors or guides and parents plays a role in the success of PMI application. These relationships thrive upon trust and transparent communication practices that foster an understanding among all parties. Unlike therapist-led interventions, which often place professionals in a position of expertise while relegating parents to recipients of knowledge and support services, the PMI acknowledges the valuable insights that parents bring to the table as experts in comprehending their children's needs and unique challenges. This recognition encourages a teamwork mindset and boosts parents' eagerness to actively participate in organized interventions grounded in science [41].

### 10.3 Clear goals lead to tangible outcomes for children

The effectiveness of PMIs is optimized when centered around goals that have an impact on enhancing a child's development. PMIs focus on enhancing aspects such as social communication skills, emotional management, and adaptive abilities, which are the primary challenges for children with autism.

### 10.4 Supporting parents' well-being for sustainable outcomes

Improving parents' well-being is crucial to the success of PMI programs aimed at enhancing child development and adjustment outcomes [42]. Factors, such as stress levels and socioeconomic background, play a role in shaping children's progress within these interventions. An efficient PMI embraces a method that incorporates strategies into parents' everyday schedules, while boosting their understanding of stress relief methods [43, 44].

### 10.5 System for sustained engagement and real-world applications

Continuous parental engagement is crucial, and interventions should be designed with the specific needs of families in mind rather than imposing rigid, one-size-fits-all models [44]. It is important for interventions to consider the unique requirements of each family rather than implementing generic solutions that may not be effective for everyone. Parents require consistent support and encouragement throughout the intervention to ensure lasting positive outcomes. Additionally, PMIs should offer structured opportunities for parents to review their progress, address difficulties, and enhance their skills gradually over time. This could be accomplished by having follow-up meetings joining support groups with peers or using platforms to maintain learning and engage with experts continuously.

### 10.6 Assessment of effectiveness and efficacy

Assessing the effectiveness and efficiency of an intervention involves monitoring both the term and long-term results to accurately determine its impact on the application of PMI. One important measure is parental treatment integrity – the extent to which parents consistently and correctly apply intervention techniques in a real-life setting. Monitoring is crucial for tracking the success of a program and refining training methods for better outcomes [45].

## 11. Types of parent-mediated autism interventions: Implementation and evidence on their effectiveness

Parent-Mediated Autism Interventions can be categorized into five major types based on their goals and focus: [1] Language and communication interventions, [2]

Behavioral-based models, [3] cognitive and socio-emotional approaches, [4] comprehensive developmental approaches, and [5] hybrid or Naturalistic Developmental Behavioral Interventions (NDBIs) (**Table 2**).

### 11.1 Language and communication-focused PMAI

Early language- and communication-focused PMIs train parents and caregivers to help their children's speech, language, and communication development through structured programs. These interventions offer benefits to children with developmental delays, autism spectrum disorder (ASD), and other communication difficulties. It has been observed that such interventions offer benefits to children facing delays or communication challenges, like autism spectrum disorder (ASD). Studies have shown that early language programs led by parents can greatly enhance a child's ability to express themselves and understand language better if started before the age of five [46]. These approaches are cost effective and adaptable across different settings. Some well-established language- and communication-focused PMIAs include the following:

- *Hanen's more than words (HMTW)*: This evidence-based program has been proven to help toddlers with autism spectrum disorder (ASD) improve their communication and social skills effectively. Caregivers are taught how to identify and react to their child's communication efforts, which, in turn, supports the child's language development during interactions [47]. Studies have shown that it is successful in enhancing both speaking and understanding abilities [5].

- *Joint attention mediated learning (JAML)*: This program was created to boost attention skills in children. This is crucial for effective interaction and communication. Research shows that JAML interventions have an impact on the engagement and verbal communication abilities of young children diagnosed on the autism spectrum [10, 48].

- *Picture exchange communication system (PECS)*: The PECS is an augmentative and alternative communication (AAC) system that teaches children with ASD to initiate communication using pictorial representations. It was developed by Bondy and Frost [49]. Flippin et al. [50] and Ganz et al. [51] have shown that ASD improves communication skills and decreases behavior in individuals with ASD.

### 11.2 Behavioral-based PMIAs

Behavioral-based PMIs train parents to use structured behavioral strategies to help improve communication skills and social interactions in children with ASD. These programs mainly draw upon the principles of Applied Behavior Analysis to encourage and decrease behavior, as shown in the research by Bearss et al. [25]. Research has also highlighted the impact of ABA-focused parent training on enhancing language abilities and social interactions while addressing challenging behaviors, according to Neimy et al. [52].

Some prominent behavior-focused PMIA examples are.

- Pivotal response treatment (PRT) focuses on aspects of development, such as motivation and social engagement. Research has indicated that when parents implement PRT, it enhances communication skills and self-initiated actions in children with ASD [4, 53].

| Target area | Program name | Age range | Description |
|---|---|---|---|
| Language & Social Communication | Hanen's *More Than Words* | Toddler | Focuses on early autism symptoms and parent-rated outcomes. |
| | Joint Attention Mediated Learning | Preschool | RCT-based program for young children with autism, emphasizing parent education. |
| | Picture Exchange Communication System (PECS) | Not specific | Increases spontaneous communication and reduces problematic behaviors by providing a reliable mode of expression. |
| Behavior-Based Interventions | Pivotal Response Training (PRT) | Young children | Includes an enhanced PRISM model. RCTs demonstrate effectiveness with no reported adverse effects. |
| | RUBI Parent Training Program | Not specified | Improves children's adaptive skills and reduces behavioral challenges, particularly when parents implement techniques with fidelity. ABA-based approaches may require high-intensity training, which some families find difficult to sustain. |
| Cognitive & Social-Emotional Focus | Parent-Child Interaction Therapy (PCIT) | Up to 13 years | Designed for managing disruptive behavior; applicable to older children. |
| | Social Stories | Not specified | Effective in improving social skills, emotional regulation, and adaptive behaviors. |
| | *The Incredible Years®* (IY) Parent Training | Not specified | Has long-term benefits in reducing conduct problems and improving emotional regulation. |
| | Responsive Teaching (RT) | Not specified | Enhances children's engagement, language acquisition, and social-emotional skills, making it beneficial for children with ASD and other developmental challenges. |
| | JASPER (Joint Attention, Symbolic Play, Engagement, & Regulation) | Not specified | Improves social communication skills and increases engagement in children with ASD. |
| Comprehensive Developmental Approaches | Child-Directed Interaction Training | Young children | Focuses on both parent and child outcomes; parent-rated effectiveness. |
| | PLAY Project Home Consultation | Young children | Includes mechanisms of developmental change with RCT evidence supporting its effectiveness. |
| | DIR/Floortime Parent Training | Preschool | Pilot RCT-based intervention focusing on preschool-aged children with ASD. |
| Hybrid or Naturalistic Developmental Behavioral Interventions (NDBIs) | Steppingstones Triple P | 2–9 years | RCT-supported parenting program aimed at reducing behavioral problems. |
| | Parent-Implemented Early Start Denver Model (P-ESDM) | Toddler | Significantly enhances language and social skills when implemented by parents. |
| | Project ImPACT | Not specified | Effective in both social-communication and behavioral domains. |

| Target area | Program name | Age range | Description |
|---|---|---|---|
| | Enhanced Milieu Teaching (EMT) | Young children | Improves expressive and receptive language skills, increases spontaneous communication, and fosters social engagement in children with language impairments. |
| | Cooperative Parent-Mediated Therapy | Preschool | Italian-based RCT intervention for preschool children with ASD. |

**Table 2.**
*Type of PMAIs.*

- RUBI parent training program: This program aims to educate parents on using behavior management strategies to decrease aggression levels and minimize tantrums and disruptive behaviors in children. Studies have indicated the effectiveness of the RUBI parent-training program [25, 54].

### 11.3 Cognitive and socio-emotional focused PMIAs

Cognitive and socio-emotional PMIs aim to enhance children's ability to effectively manage their thoughts and emotions by engaging parents in structured interventions. These interventions prioritize activities such as attention exercises alongside emotion guidance and interactive play to enhance skills and emotional control [9, 55]. Some of the evidence based PMAIs that focus on:

- Parent child interaction therapy (PCIT), which was initially developed to address distributive behaviors in children, has been modified to enhance social communication skills in children with ASD. Research indicates that PCIT does not foster parent-child bonds but also promotes better emotional control and decreases outwardly negative behaviors [48, 56].

- Social stories (ST), a program created by Carol Gray, offers narratives that support children with autism in grasping social norms better. The effectiveness of Social Stories in enhancing skills and emotional regulation has been supported by previous research [57, 58].

- Responsive teaching (RT): This program aims to support parents in nurturing their children's development and emotional well-being through attentive communication techniques. Research suggests that RT can enhance children's involvement in activities and boost their language skills and emotional development, which is beneficial for children with ASD [59, 60].

### 11.4 Comprehensive developmental approaches PMIAs

Comprehensive developmental interventions focus on holistic child development and integrating cognitive, social-emotional, and communication goals. These programs emphasize social engagement, joint attention, and play-based learning while reducing reliance on structured reinforcement techniques [61].

Some known and detailed developmental examples of PMAI have been previously reported.

- The PLAY Project is a PMI program that encourages play and has proven effective in enhancing communication skills and play habits among children with ASD [48, 56].

- The DIR/Floortime model: This program encourages parents to connect with their children through interactions to improve communication proficiency and emotional control while developing their problem-solving abilities [6, 62].

### 11.5 Hybrid or naturalistic developmental behavioral interventions (NDBIs)

NDBIs integrate principles of ABA and developmental science to create structured yet flexible interventions. These models emphasize embedded learning opportunities, natural reinforcers, and child-led interactions [39]. Research indicates that NDBIs improve language, cognitive function, and social initiation, while being feasible for community implementation [39, 56, 63].

Some types of PMAI have focused on natural developmental and behavioral interventions.

- The Parent Focused Early Start Denver Model (Parent Focused ESDM) combines ABA methods with play-based strategies to improve language abilities and cognitive development in children diagnosed with autism spectrum disorder (ASD) [64].

- Project ImPACT (Improving Parents as Communication Teachers) is a designed program that spans 16 weeks and aims to educate parents on utilizing prompting techniques and positive reinforcement along, with engaging interactions to enhance the communication and social abilities of children diagnosed with ASD (Ingersoll & Wainer 2013).

- Enhanced Milieu Teaching (EME) is a program that incorporates elements from both developmental strategies to support communication development in children experiencing language delays or ASD symptoms [65, 66]. These studies suggest that EME improves receptive language abilities, enhances social interactions, and fosters spontaneous communication in this population.

## 12. Cultural and contextual adaption in PMAIs

Effective implementation of PMIs requires cultural and contextual adaptations to the needs of a particular community [10]. PMIs have been widely recognized as an effective approach for supporting children with developmental disabilities, including autism spectrum disorders. Nevertheless, many of these interventions were initially developed in Western high-income countries, raising concerns regarding their applicability across diverse cultural and socioeconomic settings. To bridge this gap, researchers and practitioners have emphasized the need for cultural and contextual adaptations that ensure that PMIs align with the values, traditions, and daily realities of families in various communities [67].

Adapting interventions to fit cultures means adjusting them to align with the beliefs and parenting styles of various communities [68]. For example, in Latin American families, concepts such as familismo promoting close family ties and respeto emphasizing respect for authority are key factors shaping how children are raised. DuBay [69] found that interventions incorporating these values were more effective in engaging parents and sustaining long-term participation. When parents see their cultural norms reflected in an intervention, they are more likely to actively engage and apply strategies in meaningful ways.

Zeleke et al. [70] emphasized the importance of considering context in behavioral interventions, noting that parents who understand and apply behavioral principles within their cultural framework see more sustainable improvements. Functional behavioral assessments conducted by parents help identify triggers and develop personalized intervention plans that reduce maladaptive behaviors and promote positive alternatives.

In addition, to consider values and beliefs when implementing parent-mediated interventions, it is crucial to adapt them to the circumstances of families with limited financial resources adequately. Children's caregivers in low- and middle-income regions often encounter obstacles such as limitations and a lack of access to professional therapists due to the various responsibilities they juggle daily. To tackle these issues effectively, interventions should be designed with flexibility in mind, suited to the demands of life. A study by Divan et al. [67] suggested the value of community-centered delivery approaches, the involvement of paraprofessionals, and the integration of technology as a means to broaden the reach of these interventions. To enhance family engagement and maintain interest, it is helpful to incorporate PMIs into existing support networks and community settings. The Caregiver Skills Training (CST) Program by the World Health Organization is a model PMI that has been widely embraced globally. CST was developed for caregivers of children with disabilities and is cost-effective and flexible in cultural contexts. The program focused on communication skills and methods for managing emotions and behavior. It aims to help parents to incorporate these strategies into their lives [71]. With its presence, more than 30 countries are currently established. CST has been proven to boost assurance levels and enhance children's participation while improving their social communication abilities [72].

Recent research has demonstrated the benefits of culturally responsive PMIs. A mixed-methods study by Locke et al. [73] examined interventions for children with autism and found that incorporating indigenous parenting practices, alternative communication methods, and community involvement led to stronger parental engagement and better intervention outcomes. These findings suggest that when families perceive interventions as relevant to their lived experiences, they are more likely to embrace and sustain their use [68].

## 13. Key elements influencing the efficiency of PMAIs

The effectiveness of PMIs is impacted by elements such as traits of children and their parents' engagement level in the program, and the design of interventions provided in different environmental settings with support systems in place for assistance and guidance purposes that are crucial for improving outcomes and ensuring that the interventions work well for a wide range of people.

### 13.1 Factors related to children

The effectiveness of PMIs is greatly influenced by a child's age. Studies suggest that younger children below the age of seven tend to experience the advantages of PMIs due to their increased ability to learn and apply new skills early in life [61]. Introducing interventions during infancy and toddlerhood has been shown to enhance communication skills and adaptive behaviors while decreasing the severity of autism symptoms [24]. Hence, detection and intervention are crucial for optimizing the results.

Children's language abilities play a role in their responses to the PMI intervention. Those with language skills initially tend to show progress in communication and social interactions compared with those with minimal verbal capabilities [59]. Verbal children may focus on enhancing their speaking and understanding skills, while nonverbal children typically start by developing verbal communication behaviors, such as joint attention and gesturing, which form the basis for future language development [74]. Ensuring that intervention methods are customized to match a child's language proficiency is vital for fostering interaction and advancement in learning.

The level of autism symptoms can influence how well an intervention works. Kids with mild to moderate symptoms tend to improve faster in their social skills and adaptability than those with more severe symptoms, who may need more time and adjustments to see benefits from PMIs [75]. Some studies indicate that the effectiveness of PMIs does not decrease with severity but calls for personalized approaches and increased effort to achieve similar progress [76].

Regarding how PMIs work for children in need of support and intervention services, such as those with disabilities or challenges affecting their cognitive abilities and reasoning skills, higher levels of cognitive functioning play a key role in determining success rates according to studies [77]. Kids with skills are likely to benefit more from intervention approaches and apply what they learn more effectively compared to those with weaker cognitive abilities, who might require additional support strategies such as repetitive practice or visual aids to enhance their response to PMIs.

### 13.2 Parents/caregivers factors

Parental or caregiver consistency and faithfulness play a role in the effectiveness of PMIs. Research has shown that maintaining levels of fidelity, meaning carrying out intervention strategies, results in better outcomes for children's development [78]. Supporting fidelity can be achieved through expert guidance and support from professionals as consistent feedback and by following structured intervention plans to help parents feel empowered in nurturing their child's growth.

Parental education could also play a role in how PMIs are put into practice as per some research findings that indicate parents with higher levels of education tend to follow intervention guidelines more closely and have a deeper grasp of behavioral concepts that could lead to improved outcomes for children [79]. Nonetheless, ensuring that intervention resources are easy to access and culturally tailored can help connect parents from different backgrounds.

According to research by Bearss et al. [11], parental engagement plays a role in the success of PMI outcomes. When parents actively participate in implementing strategies and practicing intervention techniques with their children, they often observe enhancements in communication and adaptive skill development. Encouraging motivation and offering support can boost engagement levels and ensure continuity of interventions over an extended period.

Parental well-being is another factor that significantly affects the success of PMIs. Stress levels and mental health conditions such as depression and anxiety in parents can hinder intervention adherence and negatively impact child outcomes [80].

Conversely, when parents receive support, they show better consistency in implementing interventions, resulting in more successful outcomes [81]. Including health support for parents within PMI programs can improve both the welfare and effectiveness of interventions.

### 13.3 Intervention design

The nature and characteristics of the intervention design are other primary factors that determine its efficacy. Customizing PMIs to cater to the specific needs of children and families significantly enhances the effectiveness of interventions. Tailored interventions that consider a child's stage as well as their strengths and difficulties lead to more meaningful involvement and acquisition of skills [76]. Moreover, incorporating intervention strategies into a family's activities promotes compliance and application in various settings [53].

The length and duration of PMAI also play a role in program effectiveness [82]. Interventions that are more intense and longer lasting tend to lead to developmental results over time. However, overly intense interventions may become burdensome for families. Hinder their commitment to the program. Striking a balance between intensity and practicality is essential to ensuring participation in the run.

The delivery method of the intervention was also found to be a contributing factor to the intervention efficacy. Both face-to-face and online PMAIs have proven effective in practice. In-person coaching offers feedback and direct demonstrations to participants, and tele practice enhances access for families residing in underprivileged regions [83]. Adoptive models incorporating both in person and coaching could maximize impact while accommodating family needs effectively.

### 13.4 Environmental factors

The success of PMIs is also shaped by how families gain access to other support services such as speech therapy, occupational therapy, and inclusive educational settings [79]. Integrating different services helps to reinforce skills in different settings, leading to sustained developmental gains.

Research also shows that lower social and economic status can create obstacles for implementing PMIs due to factors such as a lack of access to resources for interventions [79]. Offering discounted interventions and adaptable program formats can help to address these inequalities. In underserved regions, families frequently encounter difficulties in accessing autism services, thus affecting the implementation and effectiveness of PMIs [54]. Telehealth interventions have risen as remedies to bridge the service gap for families isolated by geography.

Effective professional support also considers a major variable that plays a role in boosting the fidelity of PMIs and improving child outcomes over time [83]. Parents who engage in coaching and receive feedback tend to show a commitment to interventions and feel more self-assured when applying strategies. The ongoing guidance from professionals also contributes to the refinement and adjustment of intervention methods as children grow and progress.

Social connections within the community, such as parent support groups and local autism programs, are crucial for maintaining involvement in programs for children with ASD. Research indicates that peer support can help alleviate stress and build the ability to cope with challenges [81].

## 14. Emerging trends and future directions

In recent years, PMAIs have undergone significant changes as researchers are increasingly looking to enhance their accessibility and effectiveness, while also making them more culturally relevant. New trends are emerging that are shaping the future of these interventions, such as interventions, parental training through telehealth platforms, and interventions that promote parental well-being. There is also a focus on personalized approaches, cultural adaptations, and policy backing. These advancements indicate a move towards interventions that are family oriented, flexible, and scalable, with a focus on improving child outcomes and empowering parents.

### 14.1 Preemptive interventions in infancy

There has been a change in how autism intervention studies are approached, with the introduction of preventive measures that involve parents and target infants at a higher risk of autism. Similar to those with older siblings on the spectrum or showing initial signs of variance in social communication. Whitehouse and colleagues [84] carried out a controlled trial in Australia that included parents of 9-month babies displaying behaviors resembling autism who were provided with a preventive intervention program facilitated by parents themselves. By the time they turned three years old, the intervention group had significantly fewer autism traits, with only 7% meeting the ASD diagnostic criteria compared to 21% in the control group [84]. This indicates that guiding infant-parent interaction during infancy could possibly alter developmental trajectories, potentially reducing autism severity or decreasing the likelihood of a diagnosis.

Similar research conducted in both the United Kingdom (known as iBASIS) and the United States is delving into early intervention approaches aimed at improving social communication skills by emphasizing parental responsiveness, warm affect, and structured social engagement to enhance early social- communication skills before social deficits become more pronounced [24]. This study represents a paradigm shift from reactive intervention after diagnosis to preventative intervention, emphasizing the role of parents as primary mediators of early social development.

### 14.2 Telehealth and remote parent training

The rise of telehealth and distance-based parent-mediated interventions has dramatically expanded access to autism interventions. The widespread adoption of interventions has made it easier for therapists to guide parents from a distance by overcoming challenges, such as access to services based on location and transportation issues that were further exacerbated by the impact of the COVID 19 pandemic [11].

Studies with randomized controlled trials have demonstrated that offering coaching through telehealth can be as beneficial as in person therapy sessions. Koegel et al. [85] revealed that caregivers who participated in coaching in pivotal response treatment (PRT), a type of PMAI experienced notable enhancements in guiding autistic children in developing communication skills and achieved results similar to those of face, to face training sessions. Another study showed that using telehealth to teach communication skills effectively helped decrease behavior in children with autism by providing parents with tools to manage behavior [86].

Another innovative approach involves the use of AI-infused augmented reality (AR) for social-emotional learning [13]. This study introduces EMooly, an interactive

AR-based intervention that facilitates parent-child engagement through digital storytelling and gamified learning. The authors suggested that AI-based PMI interventions can enhance motivation and engagement in children with autism, making learning more interactive and adaptive to individual needs.

As research on technology-enhanced PMI progresses, it is becoming clear that digital tools can help bridge gaps in autism services, particularly for families with limited access to in-person therapy [87].

While there are advantages to telehealth services for parent training programs globally [88, 89], it is important to acknowledge the existing challenges that persist, such as access to high-speed Internet and suitable environments for remote therapy sessions and the potential difficulties in providing hands-on coaching techniques remotely. Despite these hurdles, the scalability, cost-effectiveness, and accessibility of telehealth make it a promising avenue for extending parent training interventions.

### 14.3 Parents' well-being and coaching methods

Research on PMI also considers the well-being of parents and coaching techniques as a growing area of interest. Raising a child with autism can result in excessive stress among caregivers [11]. As a result, contemporary parenting programs include components such as stress management, mindfulness practices, and parental self-care in addition to strategies that focus on the child.

Recent research indicates that using coaching methods, such as guided practice and feedback, can lead to increased involvement and improved retention of skills in the long run, compared to traditional lecture-based approaches [90]. Moreover, certain programs are now evaluating their impact on health outcomes, such as reducing stress levels, enhancing empowerment, and improving quality of life. This highlights the importance of considering well-being as an aspect of ensuring sustainable intervention.

### 14.4 Individualized and eclectic approaches

The field is now shifting away, from "one-size-fit-all" approaches towards individually tailored parent-mediated interventions. For example, in cases where a child has limited abilities and experiences levels of irritability, a parent's guidance plan could involve a mix of alternative communication methods (such as picture exchange systems) along with strategies for behavior management. Alternatively, when a child possesses skills but tends to avoid interactions, parents can concentrate on activities that promote reciprocal play and enhance social interaction [90, 91].

Roberts et al. [92] discovered that adjusting how interaction styles are tailored to match parents' natural communication tendencies resulted in improved implementation and progress for children participating in the study's intervention programs. The study's results align with the trend of integrating proven strategies from models, like applied behavior analysis (ABA) developmental play-based interventions and naturalistic developmental behavioral interventions (NDBI) to develop adaptable and personalized intervention strategies.

## 15. Conclusion

Over time, parent-led programs have become a source of encouragement for families dealing with the challenges of autism spectrum disorder (ASD). These initiatives aim to empower parents with the tools to foster their child's growth and have significantly reshaped the realm of autism intervention. Parent-mediated intervention draws from a combination of foundations such as social learning theory and applied behavior analysis to cater to the diverse requirements of children with autism.

The proof was quite convincing indeed! Research has consistently indicated that interventions facilitated by parents can positively impact communication skills and language development in children with autism, while also improving functioning and strengthening parent–child interactions. Noteworthy programs, such as the Early Start Denver Model (ESDM), Joint Attention Symbolic Play Engagement and Regulation (JASPER), and Pivotal Response Treatment (PRT), have shown enhancements in these areas. These findings support the notion that parents equipped with such tools have the potential to bring about changes in their children's lives. Apart from the data itself, its numerical representation of outcomes achieved by these interventions lies in the true significance of how they empower families to thrive and grow stronger together as a unit. Exemplified by parents' direct involvement in their child's therapy sessions, this does not enhance skill acquisition. This also leads to a boost in self-assurance and decrease in stress levels. This transformative shift from being a recipient of professional assistance to actively engaging in the process triggers a chain reaction, enabling children to apply what they have learned across various environments such as their home, school, and community.

Despite the benefits, parent-mediated interventions are not universally applicable. In this regard, cultural sensitivity plays a key role. Initiatives such as WHO Caregiver Skills Training highlight the importance of tailoring interventions to cater to backgrounds and economic situations. This flexibility is vital for addressing disparities in accessibility and involvement within marginalized communities.

The field of parent-mediated autism intervention is undergoing transformation with advancements emerging every day. Technology plays a role in reaching families that face difficulties in accessing services by offering guidance and telehealth initiatives that remove obstacles in their way of receiving help. Researchers are exploring interventions for infants at risk of developing ASD. Exploring ways to tackle issues such as anxiety from an early stage.

Challenges persist in ensuring intervention delivery methods and providing support to parents dealing with significant stress levels, while also enhancing accessibility for those who are most in need.

In general, research shows that parent-mediated interventions are becoming more crucial in treating autism, as they progress further into the future. Enhancing tailored strategies and utilizing technology for access while conducting research to grasp long-lasting effects are pivotal. By making parents central to the intervention process, PMI could enhance not only the growth of children with ASD, but also greatly impact the overall happiness of families as a whole.

## Acknowledgements

The authors acknowledge the use of Grammarly for language polishing of the manuscript.

## Author details

Waganesh A. Zeleke* and Jihad Torky
Virginia Commonwealth University, VA, USA

*Address all correspondence to: zelekew@vcu.edu

## References

[1] American Psychiatric Association. Diagnostic and Statistical Manual of Mental Disorders. 5th ed. USA: American Psychiatric Publishing; 2013

[2] Hodges H, Fealko C, Soares N. Autism spectrum disorder: Definition, epidemiology, causes, and clinical evaluation. Translational Pediatrics. 2020;**9**(Suppl 1):S55-S65. DOI: 10.21037/tp.2019.09.09

[3] Brookman-Frazee L, Vismara L, Drahota A, Stahmer A, Openden D. Parent training interventions for children with autism spectrum disorders. Behavior Modification. 2009;**33**(6):682-706

[4] Bearss K. History and theoretical foundations of parent training. In: Johnson CR, Butter EM, Lawrence S, editors. Parent Training for Autism Spectrum Disorder: Improving the Quality of Life for Children and their Families [Internet]. Washington: American Psychological Association; 2019. pp. 11-37. Available from: https://content.apa.org/books/16088-002

[5] Conrad CE, Rimestad ML, Rohde JF, Petersen BH, Korfitsen CB, Tarp S, et al. Parent-mediated interventions for children and adolescents with autism spectrum disorders: A systematic review and meta-analysis. Frontiers in Psychiatry. 2021;**12**:773604. DOI: 10.3389/fpsyt.2021.773604/full

[6] Barber AB, Swineford L, Cook C, Belew A. Effects of project ImPACT parent-mediated intervention on the spoken language of young children with autism spectrum disorder. Perspectives of the ASHA Special Interest Groups. 2020;**5**(3):573-581

[7] Siller M, Morgan L. Systematic review of research evaluating parent-mediated interventions for young children with autism: Years 2013 to 2015. In: Siller M, Morgan L, editors. Handbook of Parent-Implemented Interventions for Very Young Children with Autism. Cham: Springer International Publishing; 2018. pp. 1-21. DOI: 10.1007/978-3-319-90994-3_1

[8] Akhani A, Dehghani M, Gharraee B, Hakim SM. Parent training intervention for autism symptoms, functional emotional development, and parental stress in children with autism disorder: A randomized clinical trial. Asian Journal of Psychiatry. 2021;**62**:102735. Available from: https://linkinghub.elsevier.com/retrieve/pii/S187620182100191X

[9] Kaminski JW, Valle LA, Filene JH, Boyle CL. A meta-analytic review of components associated with parent training program effectiveness. Journal of Abnormal Child Psychology. 2008;**36**(4):567-589

[10] Green J, Charman T, Pickles A, Wan MW, Elsabbagh M, Slonims V, et al. Parent-mediated intervention versus no intervention for infants at high risk of autism: A parallel, single-blind, randomized trial. Lancet Psychiatry. 2015;**2**(2):133-140. DOI: 10.1016/S0140-6736(10)60587-9

[11] Bearss K, Burrell TL, Stewart L, Scahill L. Effect of parent training vs parent education on behavioral problems in children with autism spectrum disorder: A randomized clinical trial. JAMA. 2018;**320**(13):1327-1335. DOI: 10.1001/jama.2018.14645

[12] Diggle T, McConachie HR, Randle VR. Parent-mediated early intervention for young children with autism spectrum disorder. The Cochrane Database of Systematic Reviews.

[13] Pan C, Kuo T, Kuo F. Meta-analysis of the effectiveness of parent-mediated telehealth interventions in children with autism spectrum disorders. Research in Autism Spectrum Disorders. 2023;**107**:102209

[14] Kanner L. Autistic disturbances of affective contact. The Nervous Child. 1943;**2**(3):217-250

[15] Bettelheim B. The Empty Fortress: Infantile Autism and the Birth of the Self. New York: Free Press; 1967

[16] Rimland B. Infantile Autism: The Syndrome and its Implications for a Neural Theory of Behavior. New York: Appleton-Century-Crofts; 1964

[17] Schopler E, Brehm SS, Kinsbourne M, Reichler RJ. Effect of treatment structure on development in autistic children. Archives of General Psychiatry. 1971;**24**(5):415-421. DOI: 10.1001/archpsyc.1971.01750110027005

[18] Schopler E. Parents as co-therapists in the treatment of psychotic children. Journal of Autism and Childhood Schizophrenia. 1971;**1**(1):87-102. DOI: 10.1007/BF01537962

[19] Lovaas OI. Behavioral treatment and normal educational and intellectual functioning in young autistic children. Journal of Consulting and Clinical Psychology. 1987;**55**(1):3-9. DOI: 10.1037/0022-006X.55.1.3

[20] Lovaas OI. The "ME" Book. Baltimore: University Park Press; 1981

[21] Koegel RL, Koegel LK, Harrower JK, Carter CM. Pivotal response intervention I: Overview of approach. Journal of the Association for Persons with Severe Handicaps. 1999;**24**(3):174-185. DOI: 10.2511/rpsd.24.3.174

[22] Shields J, King M, Corbett C, Imray P. The EarlyBird program: Partnership with parents during early intervention. Autism. 2001;**5**(1):49-56. DOI: 10.1177/1362361301005001005

[23] Sussman F. More than Words: Helping Parents Promote Communication and Social Skills in Children with Autism Spectrum Disorders. Toronto, Ontario: The Hanen Centre; 1999

[24] Green J, Pickles A, Pasco G, Bedford R, Wan MW, Elsabbagh M, et al. Randomised trial of a parent-mediated intervention for infants at high risk for autism: Longitudinal outcomes to age 3 years. Journal of Child Psychology and Psychiatry. 2017;**58**(12):1330-1340. DOI: 10.1111/jcpp.12728

[25] Bearss K, Johnson C, Smith T, Lecavalier L, Swiezy N, Aman M, et al. Effect of parent training vs. parent education on behavioral problems in children with autism spectrum disorder: A randomized clinical trial. JAMA. 2015;**313**(15):1524-1533. DOI: 10.1001/jama.2015.3150

[26] Siller M, Sigman M. The behaviors of parents of children with autism predict the subsequent development of their children's communication. Journal of Autism and Developmental Disorders. 2002 Apr;**32**(2):77-89. DOI: 10.1023/a:1014884404276

[27] Rahman A, Divan G, Hamdani SU, Vajaratkar V, Taylor C, Leadbitter K, et al. Effectiveness of the parent mediated intervention for children with autism spectrum disorder in South Asia (PASS): A randomized controlled trial. The Lancet Psychiatry. 2016;**3**(2):128-136. DOI: 10.1016/S2215-0366(15)00388-0

[28] World Health Organization. Caregiver Skills Training for Families of Children with Developmental Delays or Disabilities. Switzerland: WHO; 2019

[29] Scott S, Dadds MR. Practitioner review: When parent training doesn't work theory-driven clinical strategies. Child Psychology and Psychiatry. 2009;**50**(12):1441-1450. DOI: 10.1111/j.1469-7610.2009.02161.x

[30] Weiland RF, Polderman TJ, Smit DJ, Begeer S, Van Der Burg E. No differences between adults with and without autism in audiovisual synchrony perception. Autism. 2023;**27**(4):927-937. DOI: 10.1177/13623613221121414

[31] Bowlby J. Attachment and Loss. Vol. 1. New York: Basic Books; 1969

[32] Ainsworth MDS, Blehar MC, Waters E, Wall S. Patterns of Attachment: A Psychological Study of the Strange Situation. Hillsdale (NJ): Lawrence Erlbaum; 1978

[33] Bosmans G, Van Vlierberghe L, Bakermans-Kranenburg MJ, Kobak R, Hermans D, Van IJzendoorn MH. A learning theory approach to attachment theory: Exploring clinical applications. Clinical Child and Family Psychology Review. 2022;**25**(3):591-612. DOI: 10.1007/s10567-021-00377-x

[34] Skinner BF. Science and Human Behavior. New York: Free Press; 1953

[35] Weiner B. An attributional theory of achievement motivation and emotion. Psychological Review. 1985;**92**(4):548-573

[36] Bronfenbrenner U. The Ecology of Human Development: Experiments by Nature and Design. Cambridge (MA): Harvard University Press; 1979

[37] Bowen M. Family Therapy in Clinical Practice. New York: Jason Aronson; 1985

[38] Miller WR, Rollnick S. Motivational Interviewing: Preparing People to Change Addictive Behavior. New York: The Guilford Press; 1991

[39] Schreibman L, Dawson G, Stahmer AC, Landa R, Rogers SJ, McGee GG, et al. Naturalistic developmental behavioral interventions: Empirically validated treatments for autism spectrum disorder. Journal of Autism and Developmental Disorders. 2015;**45**(8):2411-2428. DOI: 10.1007/s10803-015-2407-8

[40] Rogers SJ, Stahmer A, Talbott M, Young G, Fuller E, Pellecchia M, et al. Feasibility of delivering parent implemented NDBI interventions in low-resource regions: A pilot randomized controlled study. Journal of Neurodevelopmental Disorders. 2022;**14**(1):3. DOI: 10.1186/s11689-021-09410-0

[41] Pickard K, Hendrix N, Guerra K, Brane N, Islam N. Examining provider decisions around the delivery and adaptation of a parent-mediated intervention within an early intervention system. Autism. 2023;**27**(8):2384-2396. DOI: 10.1177/13623613231162149

[42] Shalev RA, Lavine C, Di Martino A. A systematic review of the role of parent characteristics in parent-mediated interventions for children with autism spectrum disorder. Journal of Developmental and Physical Disabilities. 2020;**32**(1):1-21. DOI: 10.1007/s10882-018-9641-x

[43] Walsh C, O'Connor P, Walsh E, Lydon S. A systematic review of interventions to improve healthcare experiences and access in autism. Review Journal of Autism and Developmental Disorders. 2023;**10**(2):185-202. DOI: 10.1007/s40489-021-00279-2

[44] Pickard KE, Kilgore AN, Ingersoll BR. Using community partnerships to

better understand the barriers to using an evidence-based, parent-mediated intervention for autism spectrum disorder in a medicaid system. American Journal of Community Psychology. 2016;**57**(3-4):391-403. DOI: 10.1002/ajcp.12050

[45] Ratliff-Black M, Therrien W. Parent-mediated interventions for school-age children with ASD: A meta-analysis. Focus on Autism and Other Developmental Disabilities. 2021;**36**(1):3-13. DOI: 10.1177/1088357620956904

[46] Pickles V, Harris J, Green C, Aldred H, McConachie VS, Charman T. Parent-mediated social communication therapy for young children with autism (PACT): Long-term follow-up of a randomized controlled trial. The Lancet. 2016;**388**(10059):2501-2509. DOI: 10.1016/S0140-6736(16)31229-6

[47] Francis G, Torgerson C, Toseeb U. Parent-mediated play based interventions to improve social communication and language skills in preschool children with autism: A systematic review and meta-analysis. Review Journal of Autism and Developmental Disorders. 2024;**17**(8)

[48] Cullenward J, Curtin M, Dos Santos V. Characteristics of effective parent-mediated interventions for parents of children with neurodevelopmental disorders in rural areas: A systematic review protocol. BMJ Open. 2024;**14**(8):e083464

[49] Bondy A, Frost L. The picture exchange communication system. Focus on Autistic Behavior. 1994;**9**(3):1-19. DOI: 10.1177/108835769400900301

[50] Flippin M, Reszka S, Watson LR. Effectiveness of the picture exchange communication system (PECS) on communication and speech for children with autism spectrum disorders: A meta analysis. American Journal of Speech-Language Pathology. 2010;**19**(2):178-195

[51] Ganz JB, Heath AK, Lund EM, Camargo SP, Rispoli MJ, Boles MB. Effects of the picture exchange communication system on communication and speech for individuals with autism spectrum disorders: A meta-analysis. American Journal of Speech-Language Pathology. 2012;**21**(2):67-80

[52] Neimy KA, Pelaez M, Carrow J. A review of parent-implemented interventions for promoting social communication skills in young children with autism spectrum disorder. Behavioral Interventions. 2020;**35**(3):350-369

[53] Koegel LK, Vernon TW, Koegel RL, Koegel BL, Paullin AW. Improving social engagement and initiations between children with autism spectrum disorder and their peers in inclusive settings. Journal of Positive Behavior Interventions. 2012;**14**(4):220-227. DOI: 10.1177/1098300712437042

[54] Nevill RE, Lecavalier L, Stratis EA. Meta-analysis of parent mediated interventions for young children with autism spectrum disorder. Autism. 2018;**22**:84-98. DOI: 10.1177/1362361316677838

[55] Landry SH, Smith KE, Swank PR. Responsive parenting: Establishing early foundations for social, communication, and independent problem-solving skills. Developmental Psychology. 2006;**42**(4):627-642

[56] Deniz E, Francis G, Torgerson C, Toseeb U. Parent-mediated play based interventions to improve social communication and language skills of preschool autistic children: A systematic review and meta-analysis. Review Journal of Autism and Developmental

Disorders. 2024;**17**(8). DOI: 10.1007/s40489-024-00463-0

[57] Gray C. The New Social Story Book. Arlington, TX, USA: Future Horizons; 2010

[58] Kokina A, Kern L. Social story™ interventions for students with autism spectrum disorders: A meta-analysis. Journal of Autism and Developmental Disorders. 2010;**40**(7):812-826

[59] Mahoney G, Perales F. Relationship-focused intervention with children with pervasive developmental disorders and other disabilities: A comparative study. Journal of Developmental and Behavioral Pediatrics. 2005;**26**(2):77-85

[60] Trivette CM, Dunst CJ, Hamby DW, O'Herin CE. Characteristics and consequences of adult learning methods and strategies. Practice Evaluation Report. 2012;**5**(1):1-32

[61] Dawson G, Rogers S, Munson J, Smith M, Winter J, Greenson J, et al. Randomized, controlled trial of an intervention for toddlers with autism: The early start Denver model. Pediatrics. 2010;**125**(1):e17-e23

[62] Greenspan SI, Wieder S. Engaging Autism: Using the Floortime Approach to Help Children Relate, Communicate, and Think. Bosten, MA, USA: Da Capo Press; 2006

[63] Chung KM, Chung E, Lee H. Behavioral interventions for autism spectrum disorder: A brief review and guidelines with a specific focus on applied behavior analysis. Journal of the Korean Academy of Child and Adolescent Psychiatry. 2024;**35**(1):29-38. DOI: 10.5765/jkacap.230019

[64] Rogers SJ, Estes A, Lord C, Vismara L, Winter J, Fitzpatrick A, et al. Effects of a brief early start Denver model (ESDM)-based parent intervention on toddlers at risk for autism spectrum disorders: A randomized controlled trial. Journal of the American Academy of Child & Adolescent Psychiatry. 2012;**51**(10):1052-1065

[65] Kaiser AP, Roberts MY. Parent implemented enhanced milieu teaching with preschool children who have intellectual disabilities. Journal of Speech, Language, and Hearing Research. 2013;**56**(1):295-309

[66] Roberts MY, Kaiser AP. Early intervention for toddlers with language delays: A randomized controlled trial. Pediatrics. 2015;**135**(4):686-693

[67] Divan G, Vajaratkar V, Cardozo P, Huzurbazar S, Verma M, Howarth E, et al. Exploring contextual adaptations in caregiver interventions for children with developmental disabilities across settings: A qualitative study. PLoS One. 2022;**17**(9):e0272077

[68] Zeleke WA, Dababnah S, Dixon P, Adere A, Reinhold Y, Hagos S, et al. Adaptation of the caregiver skills training program for Ethiopian and Eritrean immigrant families of autistic children in the US. International Journal of Developmental Disabilities. 2024:1-8. Available from: https://doi-org.proxy.library.vcu.edu/10.1080/20473869.2024.2414135

[69] DuBay M. Cultural adaptations to parent-mediated autism spectrum disorder interventions for Latin American families: A scoping review. American Journal of Speech-Language Pathology. 2022;**31**(3):1517-1534. DOI: 10.1044/2022_AJSLP-21-00239

[70] Zeleke WA, Hughes T, Chitiyo M. The path to an autism spectrum disorders diagnosis in Ethiopia: Parent perspective.

American Journal of Orthopsychiatry. 2018;**88**(3):316-327. DOI: 10.1037/ort0000249

[71] Salomone E, Pacione L, Shire S, Brown FL, Reichow B, Servili C. Development of the WHO caregiver skills training program for developmental disorders or delays. Frontiers in Psychiatry. 2019;**10**:769

[72] World Health Organization (WHO). WHO Caregiver Skills Training Programme for Families of Children with Developmental Disabilities. Switzerland; 2022

[73] Locke J, Kang-Yi CD, Pellecchia M, Mandell DS. A mixed-methods examination of culturally responsive adaptation in parent-mediated interventions for young autistic children. Administration and Policy in Mental Health and Mental Health Services Research. 2023;**50**(2):187-200

[74] Hardan AY, Gengoux GW, Berquist KL, Libove RA, Ardel CM, Phillips J, et al. A randomized controlled trial of pivotal response treatment group for parents of children with autism. Journal of Child Psychology and Psychiatry. 2015;**56**(8):884-892. DOI: 10.1111/jcpp.12354

[75] Gotham K, Pickles A, Lord C. Trajectories of autism severity in children using standardized ADOS scores. Pediatrics. 2012;**130**(5):e1278-e1284. Available from: https://publications.aap.org/pediatrics/article/130/5/e1278/32386/Trajectories-of-AutismSeverity-in-Children-Using

[76] Oono IP, Honey EJ, McConachie H. Parent-mediated early intervention for young children with autism spectrum disorders (autism spectrum disorder ASD). Cochrane Database of Systematic Reviews. 2013;**4**:CD009774. DOI: 10.1002/14651858.CD009774.pub2

[77] Anderson DK, Liang JW, Lord C. Predicting young adult outcome among more and less cognitively able individuals with autism spectrum disorders. Child Psychology and Psychiatry. 2014;**55**(5):485-494. DOI: 10.1111/jcpp.12178

[78] Stahmer AC, Rieth S, Lee E, Reisinger EM, Mandell DS, Connell JE. Training teachers to use evidence-based practices for autism: Examining procedural implementation fidelity. Psychology in the Schools. 2015;**52**(2):181-195. DOI: 10.1002/pits.21815

[79] Trembath D, Gurm M, Scheerer NE, Trevisan DA, Paynter J, Bohadana G, et al. Systematic review of factors that may influence the outcomes and generalizability of parent-mediated interventions for young children with autism spectrum disorder. Autism Research. 2019;**12**(9):1304-1321. DOI: 10.1002/aur.2168

[80] Tarver J, Palmer M, Webb S, Scott S, Slonims V, Simonoff E, et al. Child and parent outcomes following parent interventions for child emotional and behavioral problems in autism spectrum disorders: A systematic review and meta analysis. Autism. 2019;**23**(7):1630-1644. DOI: 10.1177/1362361319830042

[81] Karst JS, Van Hecke AV. Parent and family impact of autism spectrum disorders: A review and proposed model for intervention evaluation. Clinical Child and Family Psychology Review. 2012;**15**(3):247-277. DOI: 10.1007/s10567-012-0119-6

[82] Lee JD, Kang VY, Terol AK, Joo S. Examining the efficacy of culturally responsive interventions for autistic children and their families: A meta-analysis. Journal of Autism and Developmental Disorders.

2025;**55**(2):706-726. DOI: 10.1007/s10803-023-06212-2. Epub 2024 Jan 21

[83] Ingersoll B, Wainer AL, Berger NI, Pickard KE, Bonter N. Comparison of a self-directed and therapist-assisted telehealth parent-mediated intervention for children with autism spectrum disorder (ASD): A pilot RCT. Journal of Autism and Developmental Disorders. 2016;**46**(7):2275-2284. DOI: 10.1007/s10803-016-2755-z

[84] Whitehouse AJO, Varcin KJ, Alvares GA, Barbaro J, Evans K, Goodwin A, et al. Preemptive intervention versus treatment as usual for infants showing early behavioral risk signs of autism spectrum disorder: A single-blind, randomized controlled trial. The Lancet Child & Adolescent Health. 2021;**5**(11):807-817. DOI: 10.1016/S2352-4642(21)00221-8

[85] Koegel RL, Schreibman L, Good A, Cernich S, Murphy C. A randomized control trial of parent-mediated pivotal response training for children with autism spectrum disorder. Journal of Autism and Developmental Disorders. 2017;**47**(9):2768-2779

[86] Lindgren S, Wacker D, Schieltz K, Suess A, Pelzel K, Kopelman T, et al. A randomized controlled trial of functional communication training via telehealth for young children with autism spectrum disorder. Journal of Autism and Developmental Disorders. 2020;**50**(12):4449-4462. DOI: 10.1007/s10803-020-04451-1

[87] Lyu Y, Liu D, An P, Tong X, Zhang H. EMooly: Supporting autistic children in collaborative social-emotional learning with caregiver participation through interactive AI-infused and AR activities. In: Proceedings of the ACM Conference on Interactive AI for Human Interaction. 2024

[88] Fischbacher L, Dodds RL, Tien IS. Teaching parents via online asynchronous training to use speech generating devices with their autistic children: A pilot study. Children. 2024;**11**(10):1194

[89] Wainer AL, Arnold ZE, Leonczyk C, Valluripalli SL. Examining a stepped-care telehealth program for parents of young children with autism: A proof-of-concept trial. Molecular Autism. 2021;**12**(1):32. DOI: 10.1186/s13229-021-00443-9

[90] Yakubova G, Gupta S, Intepe Tingir S, Kang VY. Family-mediated interventions when teaching daily living skills to autistic individuals: A systematic review. Review Journal of Autism and Developmental Disorders. 2024

[91] Adams D, Malone S, Dargue N, Keen D, Rodgers J, Simpson K, et al. Prevention and reduction of anxiety in autistic preschoolers through an autism-specific parent-mediated intervention: A pilot randomised controlled trial evaluating short and longer term outcomes. Journal of Autism and Developmental Disorders. 2024. DOI: 10.1007/s10803-024-06570-5. [Epub ahead of print]

[92] Roberts MY, Stern YS, Grauzer J, Nietfeld J, Thompson S, Jones M, et al. Teaching caregivers to support social communication: Results from a randomized clinical trial of autistic toddlers. American Journal of Speech Language Pathology. 2023;**32**(1):115-127. DOI: 10.1044/2022_AJSLP-22-00133

Chapter 6

# Stereotypies and Self-Stimulatory Behaviors as Means of Self-Regulation in Autism

*Gerit Pfuhl and Leif Ekblad*

## Abstract

Repetitive motor behaviors, particularly stereotypies and self-stimulatory behaviors (stims), play a role in emotion- and self-regulation in autism. Less is known whether the self-regulatory function is also found in mental conditions that co-occur with autism, for example ADHD, OCD, and social phobia. In a series of online surveys, we presented stereotypy-internal state combinations. The final survey was completed by 4990 participants who indicated whether the 22 presented stereotypies were expressions of internal states for them. Participants could state (a) no diagnosis, (b) self-diagnosis, or (c) formal diagnosis of ADHD, ASD, OCD, or Social phobia. Stereotypies were done for various reasons, and various stereotypies were done for the same reason. The highest prevalence was among autistic persons, followed by persons with social phobia, OCD, and least among persons with ADHD. Co-occurrence of social phobia or OCD increased the prevalence by 1.5 stereotypy. Regarding validity, the assessed stereotypies were performed for self-regulation in autistic persons, but there was no difference in validity for persons with or without ADHD, OCD, or social phobia. Performing the stereotypy for the specific emotion was more common across all four mental conditions. Stereotypies were performed to cope with positive, negative, low, and high arousing states. There was no universal mapping of stereotypy to specific internal states. Stereotypies provide a means of self-regulation, particularly for autistic persons with co-occurring OCD or social phobia. Knowledge about the variety of human means of self-regulation can reduce the stigma of stereotypies.

**Keywords:** emotion regulation, restricted and repetitive behaviors, stimming, autistic traits, neurodiversity, communication

## 1. Introduction

What are you doing when you are bored? Taking out your smartphone and start scrolling? Without a smartphone, would you be starting to twirl your hairs, click with a pen, or fiddle with an object? These behaviors, which many of us engage in when, for example, bored, are known as stereotypies or self-stimulatory behaviors.

In the neurodiversity community, they are referred to as stims and the behavior as stimming [1]. They are a subtype of restricted and repetitive behaviors (RRB) [2]. Regarding the example of starting to scroll, the motor behavior or stereotypy of scrolling is well understood as a sign of boredom and if performed in moderation is tolerated. Excessive engagement in stereotypies, on the other hand, is problematic. In a range of mental conditions, for example autism spectrum disorder (ASD), obsessive compulsive disorder (OCD), and social phobia, the prevalence of stereotypies can be excessive and detrimental to social interactions.

This chapter reports on a cross-sectional study on the function of stereotypies across mental conditions. We refer to persons with ASD also as autistic persons.

Stereotypies are also known as stims [1]. We will not cover the development of stereotypies [3], its treatment [4], or the perception of these behaviors [5]. Our results consolidate the view that stereotypies are a means of emotion regulation and self-regulation in autistic persons. In addition, our results support that stereotypies are both reactive and proactive self-regulatory behaviors. Finally, our results reveal that comorbidities do not affect the prevalence.

### 1.1 Restricted and repetitive motor behaviors

Restricted and repetitive behaviors (RRBs) are actions or patterns of behavior that are characterized by their repetitive nature and limited range of focus. RRBs include a vast category of behaviors, ranging from restricted patterns of interest, insistence on sameness, ritualistic behaviors, compulsive behaviors, to repetitive motor manners (e.g. hand flapping) also referred to as stereotypies, and self-injurious behavior. Various subtypes have been proposed (reviewed in Ref. [2]). It is common to classify them into at least two dimensions, though most authors derived 5-6 subdomains. RRBs are often measured through interviews and observations and by using questionnaires / scales. For example, Bodfish et al. [6] found six subscales based on the Repetitive Behavior Scale-revised (RBS-R). The six subscales are: (1) Stereotyped Behavior; (2) Self-Injurious Behavior (SIB); (3) Compulsive Behavior; (4) Ritualistic Behavior; (5) Sameness Behavior; and (6) Restricted Interests Behaviors. Specifically for measuring the frequency and severity of stereotypies is the Stereotyped Behavior Scale (SBS) [7].

A recent dimensional assessment of RRBs in children and adolescents with an autism diagnosis found eight dimensions [3]; repetitive sensory motor behaviors, insistence on sameness, restricted interests, unusual interests, sensory sensitivity, self-injurious behaviors, obsessions and compulsory behaviors, and repetitive language. Obsessions and compulsory behaviors increased with age, whereas repetitive sensory motor behaviors and sensory sensitivity decreased with age. Further, they found that anxiety was positively associated with all eight behaviors.

The diagnostic and statistical manual of mental disorders-5th edition [8] has four subtypes of RRBs: (a) Stereotyped or repetitive motor movements, use of objects, or speech. (b) Insistence on sameness, inflexible adherence to routines, or ritualized patterns of verbal or non-verbal behavior. (c) Highly restricted, fixated interests that are abnormal in intensity or focus. (d) Hyper- or hyporeactivity to sensory input or unusual interests in sensory aspects of the environment [8, 9]. The subtypes are specified for ASD and note also that the subdomains are based on studies of persons with ASD.

Our study will focus on stereotypies.

### 1.2 RRBs in psychopathology

RRBs are often associated with autism spectrum disorder (ASD), but can also be observed in other mental disorders (conditions). We briefly provide an overview of RRBs in four conditions: autism, attention deficit hyperactivity disorder (ADHD), obsessive compulsive disorder (OCD), and social phobia. Our focus is on autism with the other three mental conditions viewed as prominent comorbidities.

*Autism:* Persons with an autism spectrum disorder (ASD) diagnosis and autistic persons, respectively, have differences in sensory processing, language including speech, and motor control. Restricted and repetitive motor behaviours and restricted interests are clinical diagnostic criteria for ASD [8]. Of importance, in the DSM-5, RRBs are purposeless behavior patterns that interfere with normal behaviors (see below for how outdated that view is). A recent review found that differences in the prevalence and severity of RRBs can be found from age 2 on and RRBs are reliable predictors of an ASD diagnosis between 2 and 9 years of age [10]. One study found a higher prevalence of RRBs in females compared to male autistic adolescents [11], whereas a population-based study found a higher prevalence of RRBs in male autistic persons [12]. A recent secondary data analysis of the Simons Dimplex Collection dataset showed no sex differences in repetitive and restricted behaviours and interests [13].

RRBs are generally not distressing for autistic persons [5]. However, masking is not uncommon [5, 14].

*ADHD:* RRBs are not a symptom of ADHD. ASD and ADHD often co-occur, although an ASD diagnosis often excludes an ADHD diagnosis (ICD-10). Adolescents with ADHD and RRBs show often other autistic traits too [15]. ADHD and ASD have also been linked to neuroticism and shared genetic influence [16]. We are not aware of any study measuring RRBs in ADHD. Regarding co-occurrence, studies report that from 30.6% of children diagnosed with ASD also fulfilled the criteria for ADHD [17] and up to 68.2% [18].

*OCD:* RRBs are common in OCD. Compulsive and ritualistic behaviors are a hallmark of OCD. The behavior is a means to cope with anxiety and is classified as impairing normal functioning. Patients are aware of their compulsion and obsession and RRBs are distressing for them. A recent study investigated RRBs in persons with ASD or in persons with OCD [19]. They found that the prevalence of the subtype of RRBs does differ between the two psychopathologies. Stereotypies and restricted interests are common in ASD, whereas ritualistic behaviors and compulsions are associated with OCD. Prevalence of RRBs is related to cognitive ability in ASD, whereas it is associated with inhibition, an executive function, in OCD. Further, in both psychopathologies, anxiety is a significant factor and a common comorbidity of autism [20, 21] as well as OCD [22]. Regarding comorbidity, prevalence varies from 8 to 37% [23]. Repetitive sensory motor behaviors are found in both conditions [23].

*Social phobia*: Persons with social phobia or social anxiety disorder show marked fear or anxiety about one or more social situations, for example, social interactions, being observed, and performing in front of others. The fear is disproportionate to the actual threat evoked by the social situation. Typically, persons with social phobia avoid social situations (DSM-5). Persons with a social anxiety disorder exhibit RRBs to cope with anxiety, for example fidgeting with objects. Children with this diagnosis score higher than children diagnosed with general anxiety disorder on repetitive, restricted, and stereotyped behavior [24]. Social anxiety is common in ASD, ranging from 12.9% to as high as 50% [18, 25].

In sum, no category of RRB is unique or specific to autism [26]. However, stereotypies, the focal RRB of this study, are mostly assessed in autistic persons (or their parents assess their child for that), followed by persons with social phobia and persons with OCD. Particularly in OCD, RRBs are distressing, whereas they are not solely distressing in social anxiety disorder or autism.

### 1.3 Stereotypies as a means of self-regulation

Emotions play a crucial role in helping individuals manage their thoughts, behaviors, and physiological responses to various situations. This process is known as emotional regulation, that is "individuals influence which emotions they have, when they have them, and how they experience and express them" [27]. Restricted and repetitive motor behaviors might be a means to non-verbally communicate feelings and internal states, that is a way to regulate emotions. Humans use gestures and grimaces to emphasize feelings, and humans readily attribute mental states to non-human animals and animated shapes [28, 29]. Expression and recognition of emotions regardless of the modality used facilitate normal social interaction.

To maintain a homeostatic or allostatic state one can use top-down strategies, that is redirect attention and use distraction, or bottom-up strategies, that is coping with the arousal state. Self-regulation encompasses emotion regulation but more generally refers to top-down and bottom-up processes that change emotion, behavior, or cognition to adapt to the context. It includes coping with stress and uncertainties and is a domain-general mechanism [30]. The classification into bottom-up and top-down regulatory processes should be seen along a continuum and only dichotomized for convenience. Bottom-up refers to when an external stimulus or context elicits a regulatory behavior, for example regulating being overwhelmed or excited. Top-down refers to internal mental representations that aim to achieve a state or goal, for example getting into a relaxed mood or comforting state. Proactive or top-down regulation are known to benefit mental health and increase resilience. One such beneficial strategy is cognitive reappraisal [31, 32]. Reactive strategies of self-regulation, such as suppression, avoidance, or self-harm, are seen as maladaptive [32]. Some stereotypies are self-injurious (banging head, biting, peeling, or picking cuticle or fingertip). Any excessive use of those stereotypies calls for acquiring alternative expressions. However, this should not be confused with an ideology of having to suppress RRBs [33] or using pharmacological treatments to suppress RRBs [34].

A recent study [5] on self-identified and medically diagnosed autistic persons found that stimming (expressing the stereotypies) was positive for 38%, and 56% indicating it was both positive and negative. In sum, stereotypies are means for bottom-up and top-down self-regulations, respectively.

Further, self-regulation is a process and learnable, and develops from early life to adulthood [30, 35]. Toddlers and young children show a range of self-stimulatory behaviors, but the prevalence of stereotypies reduces with aging. The reduction is slower in psychopathology, possibly due to the maturation of self-regulation and cognitive control [30].

Recent studies have investigated the function of RRBs and stereotypies, often finding them to be beneficial [5, 36, 37]. Lung et al. [36] found that stereotypies are mostly used for self-regulation, whereas insistence on sameness is mostly used to cope with anxiety, and circumscribed interests are a means for sense-making.

### 1.4 Aim of the study

Stereotypy has been measured with questionnaires, and recent studies have investigated the function and perception of stereotypies [5, 33, 38, 39]. To the best of our knowledge, no study has yet directly compared the prevalence and function (validity) of stereotypies across mental conditions, particularly those common to co-occur in autism. Recent studies on the function of stereotypies do not distinguish between proactive and reactive self-regulation strategies.

We expected a high prevalence of stereotypies in autistic persons and in persons with social phobia, a medium prevalence in persons with OCD, and a low prevalence in persons with ADHD. We expected that stereotypies function as self-regulation across diagnoses, though the strongest agreement was expected for autistic persons. Given that RRBs are common in ASD, OCD, and social phobia, but not ADHD, we expected that co-occurrence would increase the prevalence among persons with both ASD and social phobia, ASD and OCD, but not for persons with ASD and ADHD.

## 2. Methods

### 2.1 Participants

Participants were recruited from the Aspie Quiz website (www.rdos.net/eng/Aspie-quiz.php) [40]. The website is popular, attracting over 100,000 visitors per year. The website got spread in various neurodiversity fora, which explains why the proportion of persons with a diagnosis or self-diagnosis is higher than in the general population.

In phase one, 3967 participants (2438 men, 1529 women, mean age 28.64 years, sd 11.52 years) took the quiz. About 1558 scored high on neurodiversity and were offered the task. A total of 779 participants completed the stereotypy task. In the final phase, 4990 participants (2890 men, 2100 women, mean age 30.93 years, SD 14.3 years) took part. Participants could indicate whether they self-identified as an autistic person, a person with ADHD, a person with OCD, or a person having social phobia [5]. They could also state that they had a formal diagnosis for any of the four mental conditions. There was no proof of the diagnosis or interviews to confirm it. We relied on the honesty of the participants. The neurodiversity movement has contributed to a larger acceptance [41–43], and it is not uncommon that people are open about their diagnosis (e.g. the first author has yearly a handful of students telling her that they have an ASD, ADHD diagnosis, or dyslexia).

### 2.2 Ethics

Data collection was anonymous. The website clearly states that the quiz is a research tool, and data may be used for publication purposes. Proceeding meant agreeing to this term. Data collection complies with the ethical requirements for research on human subjects [44]. The study was exempt from IRB as assessed by the ethical committee at the Faculty for Social Sciences and Education, Norwegian University of Science and Technology.

### 2.3 Material: Stereotypy and internal state (SIS) task

In the first phase, we provided participants with 45 stereotypies and 32 internal states. Participants could select up to three of the 32 possible internal states for each stereotypy or "I do not do this stim" or "non-emotional reason". In this first phase, participants first took the Aspie Quiz, and only those scoring high on neurodiversity (score difference of at least 35 points) were presented with the SIS task. Table S1 provides the results. Briefly, many stims were done when bored or when thinking, and some stims were rarely done; for example, "rocking up and down" was done by 140 out of 3967 participants.

In the second phase, stereotypies were listed with four response options: (a) "I do not do this", (b) a specific reason chosen from those examined in the first phase, (c) "I do it independent of mood", and (d) "I do it for other reasons". An example is: I flap my hands when I'm excited. This was done in an iterative process to be able to find the best association between the stereotypy and internal state. To ensure validity, a few of the proposed associations were deliberately selected to be less likely. The iteration phase was first run with several incorrect associations (betaversion 9, 2006) and then in four more steps (final version 2; H20-H23, 2013). From the 45 tested stims in the first phase 17 remained, and five new ones were included after the iteration phase.

In the third and final phases, we tested 22 stereotypies and internal state pairs, plus one that served as a control, that is no known or suspected association (whistling). All visitors of the Aspie Quiz website could rate the stereotypies *before* taking the Aspie Quiz version 2. A total of 4990 volunteers completed the SIS task.

### 2.4 Procedure

The task was implemented either after volunteers took the quiz (first phase) or before they took it (second and third phases, see below). In the first phase, neurodiversity was measured based on experimental factor loadings, while in the second and third phases, Aspie Quiz final version 2 items and scoring was used. Thus, in the second and third phases, scores were consistent as the calculation was based on the same items and weight factors. The main results are based on the third and final phase where the task was implemented *before* proceeding to the Aspie Quiz. This prevented any bias in performing the task based on one's score along the neurodiverse-neurotypical continuum. Volunteers first read the consent page and if consenting were next asked a few sociodemographic factors, for example gender, age, diagnosis and self-identifying diagnosis (**Table 1**). Answering was optional. Next, the stereotypies and internal states task (SIS) was presented. Finally, the Aspie Quiz (150 items) was presented. All who completed enough items in the Aspie Quiz received their score along the ND-NT dimension and were included in the analysis. Note that participants could quit at any point, proceed to the quiz without providing any sociodemographic values, and skip the SIS task, respectively.

### 2.5 Data analysis

Descriptive analysis and plotting were done per diagnosis (ADHD, ASD, OCD and Social Phobia) and reason for stimming (see **Table 1, Figure 1**). For *prevalence,* we contrasted "I do not do it" answers with the three answers stating that one does this behavior. We expressed it as a proportion, that is the sum score of doing the behavior divided by 22.

| | Prevalence ASD | | | prevalence_ADHD | | | prevalence_OCD | | | prevalence_Social Phobia | | |
|---|---|---|---|---|---|---|---|---|---|---|---|---|
| | No diagnosis | Self-diagnosis | Formal diagnosis | No diagnosis | Self-diagnosis | Formal diagnosis | No diagnosis | Self-diagnosis | Formal diagnosis | No diagnosis | Self-diagnosis | Formal diagnosis |
| Talking to oneself—when hyperfocused | 0.82 | 0.88 | 0.86 | 0.83 | 0.88 | 0.83 | 0.83 | 0.90 | 0.84 | 0.82 | 0.89 | 0.89 |
| Walking on toes—for pleasure | 0.31 | 0.40 | 0.46 | 0.34 | 0.39 | 0.44 | 0.33 | 0.43 | 0.47 | 0.33 | 0.38 | 0.48 |
| Tapping fingers—when nervous | 0.72 | 0.79 | 0.82 | 0.74 | 0.79 | 0.78 | 0.73 | 0.81 | 0.80 | 0.73 | 0.79 | 0.82 |
| Biting lip, cheek or tongue—when anxious | 0.64 | 0.77 | 0.68 | 0.67 | 0.75 | 0.74 | 0.67 | 0.76 | 0.79 | 0.65 | 0.76 | 0.80 |
| Grinding teeth—when stressed | 0.41 | 0.55 | 0.52 | 0.44 | 0.54 | 0.58 | 0.44 | 0.53 | 0.67 | 0.43 | 0.53 | 0.60 |
| Watching spinning/blinking/glittering object—for pleasure | 0.41 | 0.61 | 0.67 | 0.47 | 0.56 | 0.62 | 0.47 | 0.61 | 0.58 | 0.46 | 0.57 | 0.60 |
| Pacing—when thinking | 0.54 | 0.70 | 0.70 | 0.58 | 0.70 | 0.70 | 0.58 | 0.70 | 0.70 | 0.57 | 0.66 | 0.74 |
| Spinning an object—for pleasure | 0.52 | 0.62 | 0.67 | 0.55 | 0.62 | 0.61 | 0.54 | 0.65 | 0.62 | 0.53 | 0.61 | 0.66 |
| Twirling hair—for pleasure | 0.38 | 0.51 | 0.47 | 0.42 | 0.47 | 0.50 | 0.41 | 0.51 | 0.57 | 0.39 | 0.49 | 0.55 |
| Pulling hairs from head/face/body—when frustrated | 0.36 | 0.46 | 0.51 | 0.40 | 0.43 | 0.43 | 0.38 | 0.46 | 0.59 | 0.37 | 0.45 | 0.54 |
| Rubbing arms or thighs—when anxious | 0.37 | 0.57 | 0.54 | 0.44 | 0.51 | 0.49 | 0.42 | 0.56 | 0.59 | 0.40 | 0.53 | 0.62 |
| Rubbing hands together—when anticipating | 0.37 | 0.53 | 0.55 | 0.43 | 0.52 | 0.45 | 0.42 | 0.52 | 0.50 | 0.41 | 0.49 | 0.60 |

| | Prevalence ASD | | | prevalence_ADHD | | | prevalence_OCD | | | prevalence_Social Phobia | | |
|---|---|---|---|---|---|---|---|---|---|---|---|---|
| | No diagnosis | Self-diagnosis | Formal diagnosis | No diagnosis | Self-diagnosis | Formal diagnosis | No diagnosis | Self-diagnosis | Formal diagnosis | No diagnosis | Self-diagnosis | Formal diagnosis |
| Flapping hands—when excited | 0.14 | 0.30 | 0.38 | 0.19 | 0.26 | 0.26 | 0.18 | 0.28 | 0.40 | 0.18 | 0.25 | 0.38 |
| Sticking tongue out—when hyperfocused | 0.20 | 0.29 | 0.35 | 0.22 | 0.29 | 0.31 | 0.22 | 0.30 | 0.32 | 0.21 | 0.28 | 0.32 |
| Pressing eyes—when stressed | 0.35 | 0.53 | 0.48 | 0.40 | 0.50 | 0.49 | 0.40 | 0.50 | 0.58 | 0.38 | 0.49 | 0.54 |
| Clenching and unclenching fists—when angry | 0.39 | 0.54 | 0.58 | 0.42 | 0.55 | 0.51 | 0.43 | 0.53 | 0.57 | 0.41 | 0.51 | 0.57 |
| Rocking back and forth—for comfort | 0.31 | 0.49 | 0.54 | 0.36 | 0.47 | 0.48 | 0.35 | 0.49 | 0.56 | 0.33 | 0.47 | 0.62 |
| Jumping up and down—when happy | 0.18 | 0.31 | 0.41 | 0.21 | 0.30 | 0.32 | 0.22 | 0.29 | 0.36 | 0.22 | 0.26 | 0.35 |
| Biting oneself—when anxious | 0.16 | 0.28 | 0.31 | 0.20 | 0.26 | 0.26 | 0.19 | 0.29 | 0.32 | 0.18 | 0.26 | 0.37 |
| Banging head—when upset | 0.12 | 0.22 | 0.27 | 0.15 | 0.21 | 0.24 | 0.15 | 0.23 | 0.27 | 0.14 | 0.21 | 0.25 |
| Crossing arms—when in closed state of mind | 0.68 | 0.79 | 0.73 | 0.71 | 0.79 | 0.73 | 0.71 | 0.79 | 0.78 | 0.69 | 0.77 | 0.80 |
| Pulling grass—pretending to be uninterested | 0.36 | 0.48 | 0.48 | 0.40 | 0.47 | 0.43 | 0.39 | 0.48 | 0.54 | 0.38 | 0.46 | 0.52 |
| Whistling (control stimulus) | 0.43 | 0.43 | 0.46 | 0.42 | 0.48 | 0.46 | 0.42 | 0.46 | 0.50 | 0.43 | 0.43 | 0.46 |

**Table 1.**
*The tested stereotypy-emotion pairs and their prevalence (percentage) across the four mental conditions.*

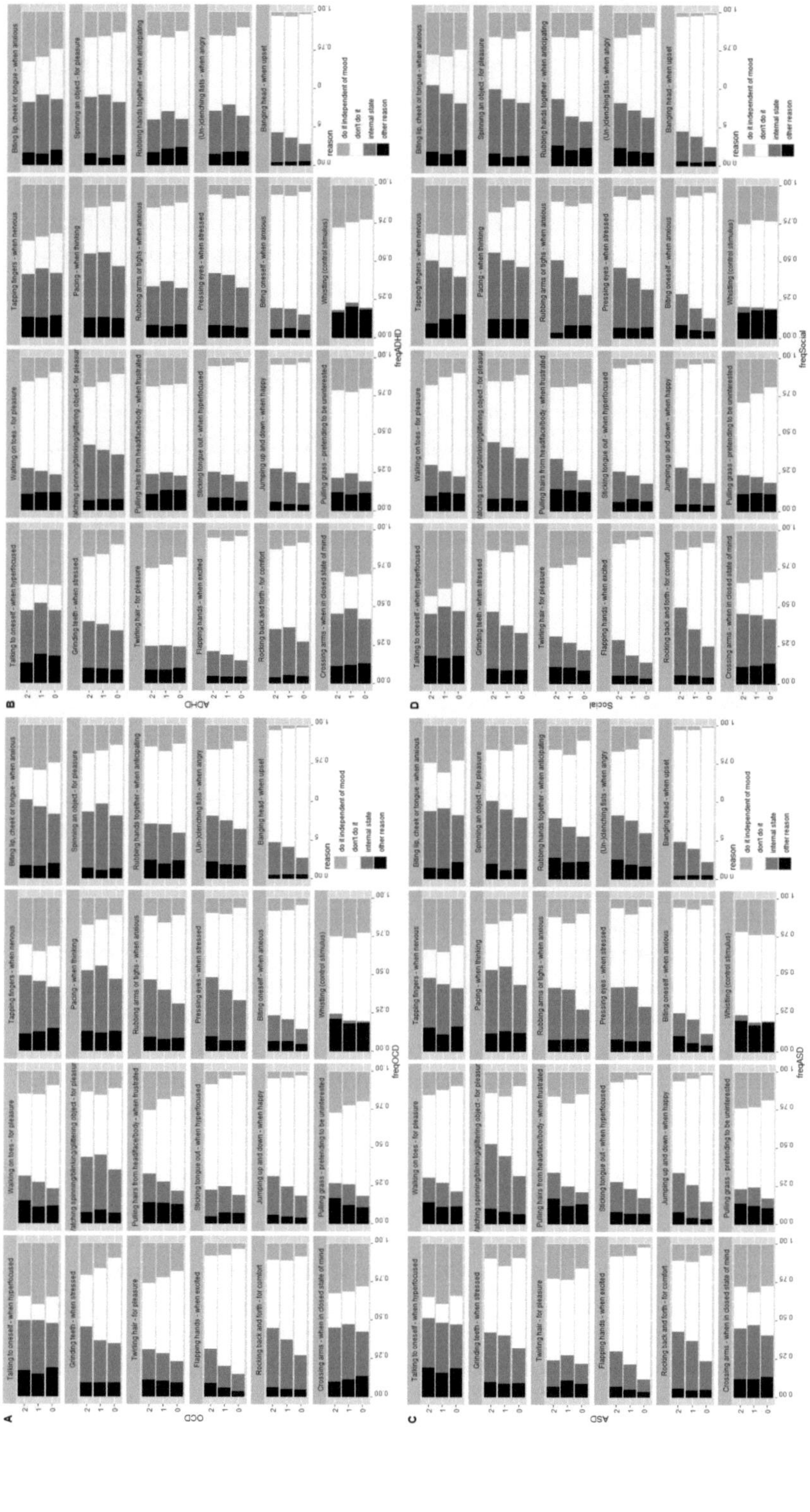

**Figure 1.**
*Barplots showing percentagewise the reason why a stereotypy is performed or not, across the four mental conditions. The control stereotypy "whistling" is also included.*

Secondly, we contrasted the option of "I do it independent of mood" with the two internal state answer options "I do it for this reason" and "I do it for another reason". We expressed it as a relative proportion, that is the sum score of doing it for self-regulation divided by the prevalence. For example, if a participant was doing 10 stereotypies, and 8 of them were for self-regulation, the score would be .8. We refer to this as validity analysis.

Thirdly, to measure how representative the chosen internal state "I do it for another reason" was, we contrasted it with "I do it for this reason" after excluding "I do not do it" and "I do it independently of mood" answers. We expressed it as a relative proportion, that is the sum score of doing it for this reason divided by the number of doing it for self-regulation. For example, if a participant was doing eight stereotypies for self-regulation, and four for the proposed emotion, the score would be .5. We refer to this as agreement analysis.

For all three analyses, we used the non-parametric Kruskal-Wallis test due to violations of assumptions that could not be rectified by transforming the outcome variable. The predictors were the four conditions, each having three levels: no diagnosis, self-diagnosis and formal medical diagnosis. We performed Dunn's post-hoc comparisons for significant conditions.

Analysis was done in R [45] and JASP [46]. The study was not pre-registered, but all material and analysis can be found at osf.io/kqd8j.

## 3. Results

### 3.1 Selection of stereotypies

In phase one, 3967 participants took the survey. Of those, 1558 had a neurodiversity score above the cutoff point and were asked to take the SIS task. A total of 797 participants continued and provided ratings of stims and internal states. Many indicated talking to oneself, and most do it when thinking. Flapping hands was reported by 373 participants, and most do it when excited. Overall, in phase 1 we found that 20 different stims were done when thinking, and 22 stims were done when bored. This illustrates that there is rarely a one-to-one mapping of stims to internal states. Furthermore, some stims were done for seemingly contradictory reasons; that is, rocking back-and-forth was done when thinking, to comfort, when overwhelmed, when overstimulated, to calm oneself, but also when distressed, when upset and when sad. Stereotypies were done for over-arousal (when anxious, when overstimulated) and under-arousal (when bored), but not for being tired or being sick. This aligns well with the study by Morris et al. [5].

To account for 50% of the answers for the preferred internal state, on average 4.6 internal states had to be selected. For 80%, on average 11.4 internal states had to be selected and for 90%, on average 16.0 internal states were required. This meant that answers were not just random. Since some of the internal states were associated with many stims (especially thinking and bored), there might be two reasons for stimming: a generic one and a specific one. Stims that mostly appeared to relate to generic reasons, and for which no specific reason could be found, were excluded from testing in phases 2 and 3. During the iteration, new stims and new internal states were evaluated. The final phase used 22 stims, 17 from phase one and 5 from the iteration phase. The tested stereotypy-emotion pairs are presented in **Table 1**, and they cover positive and negative valence, as well as low and high arousal.

There were five stereotypy-emotion pairs that were "top-down" or proactive; for example, doing the stereotypy "for pleasure", "for comfort" and 16 stereotypies could be classified as using bottom-up or reactive processes (all starting with "when"). "Pretending to be uninterested" was ambiguous and may be both top-down and bottom-up.

### 3.2 Descriptives for final phase

Among the 4990 participants, 229 reported being diagnosed with ASD (4.6%), and 1915 (38.4%) chose self-diagnosis. A total of 459 (9.2%) reported being diagnosed with ADHD, and 803 (16.1%) chose self-diagnosis. A total of 205 (4.1%) persons reported being diagnosed with OCD, and 951 (19.1%) chose self-diagnosis. A total of 282 (5.7%) reported being diagnosed with social phobia, and 1582 (31.7%) chose self-diagnosis.

Regarding comorbidities of ASD with one of the three other diagnoses, 63 (1.3%) persons reported a diagnosis of ASD and ADHD. If one includes self-diagnosis for one or both of the diagnoses, then 840 persons (16.8%) reported having both ASD and ADHD. Twenty-seven (.5%) persons report being diagnosed with both ASD and OCD. Including self-diagnosis, comorbidity of OCD with ASD was 15.2% (757 persons). Finally, ASD and social phobia were prevalent in 38 persons (.8%), including self-diagnosis in 27% (1212 persons).

### 3.3 Prevalence, validity and agreement

The overall prevalence of stereotypies was statistically significantly higher in persons indicating having a diagnosis of ASD, ADHD, OCD or social phobia, as well as among self-diagnosed persons (**Table 2**). Dunn's post hoc test found a difference between persons without ASD and self-diagnosed persons ($z = -18.84$, $p_{Holm} < .001$), and diagnosed persons ($z = -9.148$, $p_{Holm} < .001$) but not between self-diagnoses and diagnosed persons ($z = -1.023$, $p_{Holm} = .306$). Similarly, Dunn's post hoc test found a difference between persons without ADHD and self-diagnosed persons ($z = -8.35$, $p_{Holm} < .001$) and diagnosed persons ($z = -5.935$, $p_{Holm} < .001$) but not between self-diagnosed and diagnosed persons ($z = .536$, $p_{Holm} = .591$). Dunn's post hoc test found a difference between persons without OCD and self-diagnosed persons ($z = -11.65$, $p_{Holm} < .001$) and diagnosed ($z = -10.452$, $p_{Holm} < .001$) but not between self-diagnosed and diagnosed persons ($z = -1.626$, $p_{Holm} = .104$). Dunn's post hoc test found a difference between persons without social phobia and self-diagnosed persons

| | | | | | 95% CI for Rank $\varepsilon^2$ | |
|---|---|---|---|---|---|---|
| **Factor** | **Statistic** | **df** | **p** | **Rank $\varepsilon^2$** | **Lower** | **Upper** |
| ASD | 390.670 | 2 | < .001 | 0.078 | 0.064 | 0.094 |
| ADHD | 93.014 | 2 | < .001 | 0.019 | 0.013 | 0.028 |
| OCD | 177.923 | 2 | < .001 | 0.036 | 0.027 | 0.045 |
| Social phobia | 217.776 | 2 | < .001 | 0.044 | 0.034 | 0.054 |

*Note. Tests are conducted separately for each variable, without accounting for multivariate effects.*

**Table 2.**
*Prevalence of stereotypy across mental conditions.*

(z = -12.015, $p_{Holm}$ < .001) and diagnosed persons (z = -10.452, $p_{Holm}$ < .001) and also between self-diagnosed and diagnosed persons (z = -4.319, $p_{Holm}$ < .001). Thus, in all four conditions, but particularly in ASD and social phobia (based on effect size), the 22 tested stereotypies are common. The lowest prevalence was in ADHD.

Doing the stereotypy for self-regulation (validity assessment) was statistically significant for the ASD group (**Table 3**), but not for any of the other three conditions. Dunn's post hoc test found a significant difference between persons without a diagnosis and those self-diagnosed (z = 2.644, $p_{Holm}$ = .008). There was no significant difference between persons without a diagnosis and those being diagnosed (z = -.757, $p_{Holm}$ = .449) or between self-diagnosed and diagnosed persons (z = -1.861, $p_{Holm}$ = .063). Thus, performing a stereotypy for self-regulation was common among persons with ASD, but not for any of the other three conditions.

Regarding stereotypy-suggested emotion agreement, this was statistically significantly higher in persons indicating having a diagnosis of ASD, ADHD, OCD or social phobia, as well as among self-diagnosed persons (**Table 4**). Dunn's post hoc test found a significant difference between persons without an ASD diagnosis and self-diagnosed (z = -8.924, p < .001) and diagnosed persons (z = -2.804, $p_{Holm}$ = .005) but not between self-diagnosed and diagnosed persons (z = 1.018, $p_{Holm}$ = .309). The pattern was similar for ADHD, OCD and social phobia. Dunn's post hoc test found a significant difference between persons without an ADHD diagnosis and self-diagnosed (z = -4.171, $p_{Holm}$ < .001) and diagnosed persons (z = -3.689, $p_{Holm}$ < .005) but not between self-diagnosed and diagnosed persons (z = .0345, $p_{Holm}$ = .73). Dunn's post hoc test found a significant difference between persons without an OCD diagnosis and self-diagnosed (z = -5.522, $p_{Holm}$ < .001) and diagnosed persons (z = -3.066, $p_{Holm}$ = .002) but not between self-diagnosed and diagnosed persons (z = .0257, $p_{Holm}$ = .797). Dunn's post hoc test found a significant difference between persons without a social phobia diagnosis and self-diagnosed (z = -5.6, $p_{Holm}$ < .001) and diagnosed persons (z = -4.49, $p_{Holm}$ < .001) but not between self-diagnosed and diagnosed persons (z = -1.646, $p_{Holm}$ = .1). Thus, if a person is performing the stereotypy for self-regulation, it is for the suggested emotion and internal states, respectively.

### 3.4 Co-occurrence of ASD with ADHD, OCD or social phobia

Next, we investigated whether persons with a co-occurrence of ASD and OCD, ASD and social phobia, or ASD and ADHD differed in their prevalence and validity of the stereotypies. We pooled self-diagnosed and formally diagnosed as they (see above) had similar prevalence and validity. This yielded 840 participants in the group

| | | | | | 95% CI for Rank $\varepsilon^2$ | |
|---|---|---|---|---|---|---|
| **Factor** | **Statistic** | **df** | **p** | **Rank $\varepsilon^2$** | **Lower** | **Upper** |
| ASD | 8.513 | 2 | 0.014 | 0.002 | $3.059 \times 10^{-4}$ | 0.005 |
| ADHD | 4.198 | 2 | 0.123 | $8.414 \times 10^{-4}$ | $8.613 \times 10^{-5}$ | 0.003 |
| OCD | 4.766 | 2 | 0.092 | $9.553 \times 10^{-4}$ | $7.782 \times 10^{-5}$ | 0.004 |
| Social phobia | 4.119 | 2 | 0.128 | $8.256 \times 10^{-4}$ | $6.811 \times 10^{-5}$ | 0.003 |

*Note. Tests are conducted separately for each variable, without accounting for multivariate effects.*

**Table 3.**
*Kruskal-Wallis test for validity (is stereotypy done for self-regulation).*

| | | | | | 95% CI for Rank $\varepsilon^2$ | |
|---|---|---|---|---|---|---|
| **Factor** | **Statistic** | **df** | **p** | **Rank $\varepsilon^2$** | **Lower** | **Upper** |
| ASD | 81.268 | 2 | < .001 | 0.016 | 0.010 | 0.024 |
| ADHD | 27.243 | 2 | < .001 | 0.005 | 0.003 | 0.011 |
| OCD | 36.864 | 2 | < .001 | 0.007 | 0.003 | 0.013 |
| Social phobia | 44.367 | 2 | < .001 | 0.009 | 0.005 | 0.015 |

*Note. Tests are conducted separately for each variable, without accounting for multivariate effects.*

**Table 4.**
*Kruskal–Wallis test for agreement (is the stereotypy done for the suggested internal state / emotion).*

"ASD and ADHD", 757 in the group "ASD and OCD", and 1212 in the group "ASD and Social phobia".

Persons with both ASD and ADHD performed on average 12.12 (SD = 5.17) stereotypies, persons with ASD but no ADHD did on average 11.32 (SD = 5.11) stereotypies, whereas persons with neither ASD nor ADHD did on average 8.76 (sd = 4.66) stereotypies. This difference was significant, $F(2, 4987) = 219.84$, $p < .001$, $\eta^2 = .081$. All three post hoc tests were significant, that is $p < .001$; however, the effect size for the ASD only versus the ASD and ADHD group was small, Cohen's d = .163, compared to the other two effect sizes (.69 and .526). There was no difference in validity between the three groups, Kruskal-Wallis test = 5.496, p = .064.

Persons with both ASD and OCD did on average 12.69 (SD = 5.11) stereotypies, persons with ASD but no OCD did on average 11.06 (SD = 5.07) stereotypies, whereas persons with neither ASD nor OCD did on average 8.76 (SD = 4.66) stereotypies. This difference was significant, $F(2, 4987) = 242.59$, $p < .001$, $\eta^2 = .089$. All three post hoc tests were significant, that is $p < .001$. The effect sizes were Cohen's d = .337 for the ASD but no OCD versus ASD and OCD group comparison, Cohen's d = -.474 for the ASD only versus neither ASD nor OCD group, and Cohen's d = -.811 for the ASD and OCD versus neither ASD nor OCD group comparison. Thus, people with ASD and OCD do more stereotypies than persons who only have ASD.

There was no difference in validity between the three groups, Kruskal-Wallis test = 5.154, p = .076.

Persons with both ASD and social phobia did on average 12.26 (SD = 5.07) stereotypies, persons with ASD but no social phobia did on average 10.82 (SD = 5.13) stereotypies, whereas persons with neither ASD nor social phobia did on average 8.76 (SD = 4.66) stereotypies. This difference was significant, $F(2, 4987) = 237.79$, $p < .001$, $\eta^2 = .087$. All three post hoc tests were significant, that is $p < .001$. The effect sizes were Cohen's d = .298 for the ASD but no social phobia versus ASD and social phobia group comparison, Cohen's d = -.424 for the ASD only versus neither ASD nor social phobia group, and Cohen's d = -.722 for the ASD and social phobia versus neither ASD nor social phobia group comparison. Thus, people with ASD and social phobia perform more stereotypies than persons who only have ASD.

There was no difference in validity between the three groups, Kruskal-Wallis test = 5.102, p = .078.

Overall, the results align with theoretical predictions; that is, ADHD as comorbidity is only very little increasing the number of stereotypies (.8 stereotypy), whereas OCD and social phobia do increase the number of performed stereotypies to a larger extend (1.5 stereotypies more for social phobia and OCD). The function of the stereotypies is

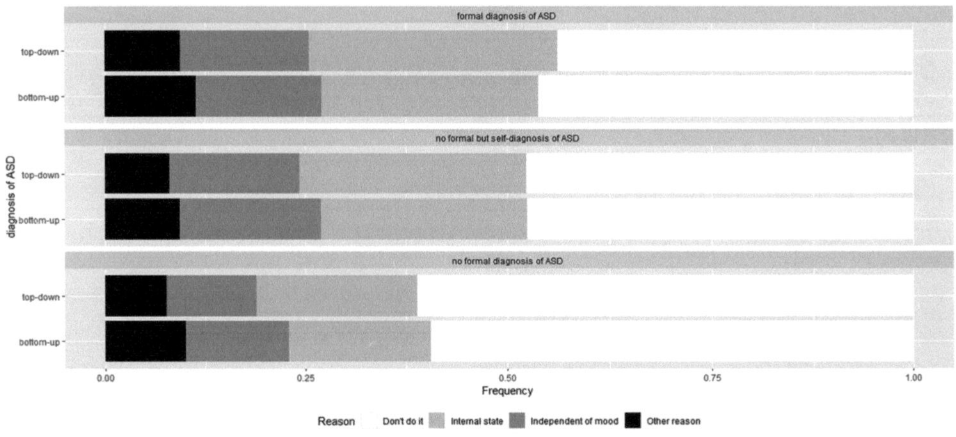


**Figure 2.**
*Barplots showing prevalence of proactive vs reactive strategies among persons w/wo autism.*

unaffected by co-occurrence; that is, the percentage of participants doing it for self-regulation was independent of the mental condition(s) a participant has.

### 3.5 Proactive versus reactive self-regulation strategies

Finally, we compared top-down with bottom-up processes, that is whether a stereotypy was proactive, that is to achieve a state of mind or whether it was reactive, that is done to cope with a, often negative, feeling in the ASD group. This was based on only this group significantly performing stereotypies for self-regulation.

A bottom-up or reactive process was conveyed by using expressions starting with "when". There was a significant overall difference between proactive and reactive processes, with stereotypies being more often done for the proposed proactive internal state than for the reactive internal state, Cochran-Mantel-Haenszel test, $\chi^2(df = 3) = 161.82$, $p < .001$. There was a higher prevalence and validity for top-down pairs than for bottom-up pairs, most pronounced among persons with a formal diagnosis of ASD (**Figure 2**). Thus, stereotypies are not non-functional behaviors, but are self-regulatory behaviors to reduce negative emotions and achieve positive emotions.

## 4. Discussion

We found 22 stereotypies that were done for a wide range of emotions, such as being nervous, anxious, stressed, frustrated, angry, and upset, but also when anticipating, when excited, for pleasure, and for comfort. This aligns with earlier findings of stereotypies being a means of regulating arousal [35] and self-regulation [5, 36, 38].

We found that stereotypies are most prominent in ASD and that a co-occurrence with social phobia or OCD increases the number of performed stereotypies. This aligns with recent findings that comorbidity with OCD or anxiety increases the intensity of restricted and repetitive motor behaviors [23].

Our study also replicated previous results of stereotypies expressing and coping with positive and negative internal states. Novel is the analysis of proactive and reactive regulatory processes. On the one hand, our iterative process kept mostly reactive processes, that is a stereotypy was done to cope with an external (bottom-up) stimulus. On the other hand, the two proactive processes, "for pleasure" and "for comfort", were associated across participants with the same four plus one stereotypies; that is, these specific stereotypies were more commonly done for pleasure/comfort, whereas the other stereotypies were more likely done for other reasons and independent of mood, respectively. Qualitative studies also report on the beneficial effect of stimming [5, 33, 39]. Notably, we found that autistic persons performed the stereotypies more often for self-regulation than persons without ASD, but there was no significant difference for persons with or without ADHD, with or without OCD, or with or without social phobia. Notably, when including co-occurrence none of the three autism-other mental disorder groups had a significant difference in validity compared to persons without any mental condition of only being autistic. This suggests that stereotypies are mostly self-regulatory for autistic persons, but persons with other mental conditions and without any diagnosis do them more for non-self-regulatory reasons. It is conceivable that not all participants consider, for example sensory regulation or avoidance behavior as mood (i.e. we formulated it as "doing it independent of mood"). A qualitative study may shed more light on the other reasons.

Across all four mental conditions agreement with the proposed mental state or emotion, respectively, was higher than in participants without a mental condition. That might be due to our stimulus selection process, that is in phase 1, only participants that scored high on neurodiversity could take the task. Still, the iterative process added five more stereotypy-emotion pairs. Previous research has also reported similarities in the reason for performing repetitive motor behaviors [35], though we are not aware of a study of stereotypies specifically in adult neurotypical persons.

Further, we found more agreement for stereotypies paired with proactive processes than for stereotypies paired with reactive processes. This might be due to heterogeneity in the means of self-regulation [5, 36] or our iterative process. Still, this is worth following up, not least given the beneficial effects of proactive self-regulatory strategies on well-being and motivation [30, 33, 47, 48].

## 5. Limitations

We recruited from a popular website, suggesting that most participants are high-functioning and fluent in English. We have no verification of their diagnosis as this was neither practical nor the primary focus of the website. We could have used a dimensional approach by using the neurodiversity-neurotypical continuum [40, 43]; however, using mental conditions allowed exploring the co-occurrence pattern. Using a neurodiversity score does not have subdimensions of OCD, ADHD or social phobia. And the autism quotient does not measure the same traits in persons with and without ASD [49].

We cannot distinguish whether stereotypies are unintentional emotional expressions or whether they are intentionally done to communicate one's emotional state [5, 33, 50]. A high prevalence of stereotypies was found in 10 persons with low-functioning ASD, a group expressing their internal states more non-verbally than verbally [50]. In these 10 individuals, many of those stereotypies were related to stress and anxiety. This aligns with our data and other research finding that RRBs become more prevalent with increasing anxiety [3, 35].

We did not assess how often participants perform the stereotypy, in which context, and whether they rated performing it as beneficial. Given that the reason (validity) for performing the stereotypy was similar across participants, future studies should investigate whether persons with and without a mental condition differ on those dimensions. It would also be relevant whether persons with and without a mental condition understand the reason for the stereotypy similarly. Far too little research has been done here, as the focus was too much on suppressing RRBs. A recent phenomenological self-investigation in autistic persons found that social misperception is likely contingent on specific contexts and interactions and not unique to autism [43].

Two stereotypies could be performed for the same emotional state, preventing unambiguous mapping of a stereotypy to an internal state. Furthermore, we cannot say whether stereotypies are generational, cultural or purely individual differences.

## 6. Conclusions

Stereotypies or stims are common in persons with ASD, OCD, social phobia and ADHD. Prevalence increased for autistic persons with a co-occurrence of any of the other mental conditions. Self-regulation was common in autism. Stereotypies serve both to regulate and react to negative feelings as well as to achieve positive feelings proactively.

## Acknowledgements

We thank all the visitors of the Aspie quiz, who contributed with their responses to studying the function of stereotypies.

## Conflict of interest

The authors declare no conflict of interest.

## Notes/thanks/other declarations

We thank Robert Biegler and Francesca Parisi for fruitful discussions on earlier versions of the manuscript.

## Author details

Gerit Pfuhl[1]* and Leif Ekblad[2]

1 Department of Psychology, NTNU, Trondheim, Norway

2 Lund University, Lund, Sweden

*Address all correspondence to: gerit.pfuhl@ntnu.no

## References

[1] Nolan J, McBride M. Embodied semiosis: Autistic 'stimming' as sensory praxis. In: Trifonas PP, editor. International Handbook of Semiotics. Dordrecht: Springer Netherlands; 2015. pp. 1069-1078

[2] Berry K, Russell K, Frost K. Restricted and repetitive Behaviors in autism Spectrum disorder: A review of associated features and presentation across clinical populations. Current Developmental Disorders Reports. 2018;**5**(2):108-115

[3] Uljarević M, Spackman EK, Whitehouse AJO, Frazier TW, Billingham W, Condron P, et al. Arriving at the empirically based conceptualization of restricted and repetitive behaviors: A systematic review and meta-analytic examination of factor analyses. Clinical Psychology Review. 2023;**103**:102286

[4] Loftin RL, Odom SL, Lantz JF. Social interaction and repetitive motor behaviors. Journal of Autism and Developmental Disorders. 2008;**38**(6):1124-1135

[5] Morris IF, Sykes JR, Paulus ER, Dameh A, Razzaque A, Esch LV, et al. Beyond self-regulation: Autistic experiences and perceptions of stimming. Neurodiversity. 2025;**3**:27546330241311096

[6] Bodfish JW et al. Varieties of repetitive behavior in autism: comparisons to mental retardation. Journal of Autism and Developmental Disorders. 2000;**30**(3):237-243

[7] Rojahn J, Matlock ST, Tassé MJ. The stereotyped behavior scale: Psychometric properties and norms. Research in Developmental Disabilities. 2000;**21**(6):437-454

[8] American Psychiatric A, Force DSMT, American Psychiatric Association P. Diagnostic and statistical manual of mental disorders : DSM-52017. In: Diagnostic and statistical manual of mental disorders: DSM-5™. 5th ed. Arlington, VA, US: American Psychiatric Publishing, Inc.; 2013

[9] Hodges H, Fealko C, Soares N. Autism spectrum disorder: Definition, epidemiology, causes, and clinical evaluation. Translational Pediatrics. 2020;**9**(Suppl. 1):S55-s65

[10] Chaxiong P, Dimian AF, Wolff JJ. Restricted and repetitive behavior in children with autism during the first three years of life: A systematic review. Frontiers in Psychology. 2022;**13**:986876

[11] Wodka EL, Parish-Morris J, Annett RD, Carpenter L, Dillon E, Michaelson J, et al. Co-occurring attention-deficit/hyperactivity disorder and anxiety disorders differentially affect males and females with autism. The Clinical Neuropsychologist. 2022;**36**(5):1069-1093

[12] Uljarević M, Cooper MN, Bebbington K, Glasson EJ, Maybery MT, Varcin K, et al. Deconstructing the repetitive behaviour phenotype in autism spectrum disorder through a large population-based analysis. Journal of Child Psychology and Psychiatry. 2020;**61**(9):1030-1042

[13] Jasim S, Perry A. Repetitive and restricted behaviors and interests in autism spectrum disorder: Relation to individual characteristics and mental health problems. BMC Psychiatry. 2023;**23**(1):356

[14] Wiskerke J, Stern H, Igelström K. Camouflaging of repetitive movements in autistic female and transgender adults. bioRxiv. 2018:412619 [Preprint]

[15] Martin J, Hamshere ML, O'Donovan MC, Rutter M, Thapar A. Factor structure of autistic traits in children with ADHD. Journal of Autism and Developmental Disorders. 2014;**44**(1):204-215

[16] Park SH, Guastella AJ, Lynskey M, Agrawal A, Constantino JN, Medland SE, et al. Neuroticism and the overlap between autistic and ADHD traits: Findings from a population sample of young adult Australian twins. Twin Research and Human Genetics. 2017;**20**(4):319-329

[17] Leyfer OT, Folstein SE, Bacalman S, Davis NO, Dinh E, Morgan J, et al. Comorbid psychiatric disorders in children with autism: Interview development and rates of disorders. Journal of Autism and Developmental Disorders. 2006;**36**(7):849-861

[18] Salazar F, Baird G, Chandler S, Tseng E, O'sullivan T, Howlin P, et al. Co-occurring psychiatric disorders in preschool and elementary school-aged children with autism Spectrum disorder. Journal of Autism and Developmental Disorders. 2015;**45**(8):2283-2294

[19] Jiujias M et al. Restricted, repetitive behaviors in autism spectrum disorder and obsessive-compulsive disorder: A comparative review. Child Psychiatry & Human Development. 2017;**48**(6):944-959

[20] Keshavarz S, Esmaeilpour K. Relationship between social anxiety and separation anxiety symptoms with insistence on sameness with the mediating role of sensory hypersensitivity. BMC Psychology. 2025;**13**(1):62

[21] Bellini S. Social skill deficits and anxiety in high-functioning adolescents with autism Spectrum disorders. Focus on Autism and Other Developmental Disabilities. 2004;**19**(2):78-86

[22] Crino RD, Andrews G. Obsessive-compulsive disorder and axis I comorbidity. Journal of Anxiety Disorders. 1996;**10**(1):37-46

[23] Brennan J et al. A systematic review of family accommodation in autistic youth: Anxiety disorders, obsessive-compulsive disorder, and restricted and repetitive behaviors. Journal of Autism and Developmental Disorders. 2025. DOI: 10.1007/s10803-025-06750-x

[24] Halls G, Cooper PJ, Creswell C. Social communication deficits: Specific associations with social anxiety disorder. Journal of Affective Disorders. 2015;**172**:38-42

[25] Montaser J, Umeano L, Pujari HP, Nasiri SMZ, Parisapogu A, Shah A, et al. Correlations between the development of social anxiety and individuals with autism spectrum disorder: A systematic review. Cureus. 2023;**15**(9):e44841

[26] Lewis M, Kim SJ. The pathophysiology of restricted repetitive behavior. Journal of Neurodevelopmental Disorders. 2009;**1**(2):114-132

[27] Gross JJ. The emerging field of emotion regulation: An integrative review. Review of General Psychology. 1998;**2**(3):271-299

[28] Castelli F, Frith C, Happe F, Frith U. Autism, Asperger syndrome and brain mechanisms for the attribution of mental states to animated shapes. Brain. 2002;**125**:1839-1849

[29] Olsson A, Ochsner KN. The role of social cognition in emotion. Trends in Cognitive Sciences. 2008;**12**(2):65-71

[30] Nigg JT. Annual research review: On the relations among self-regulation, self-control, executive functioning, effortful control, cognitive control, impulsivity, risk-taking, and inhibition for developmental psychopathology. Journal of Child Psychology and Psychiatry. 2017;**58**(4):361-383

[31] Wang K, Goldenberg A, Dorison CA, Miller JK, Uusberg A, Lerner JS, et al. A multi-country test of brief reappraisal interventions on emotions during the COVID-19 pandemic. Nature Human Behaviour. 2021;**5**(8):1089-1110

[32] Hu T, Zhang D, Wang J, Mistry R, Ran G, Wang X. Relation between emotion regulation and mental health: A meta-analysis review. Psychological Reports. 2014;**114**(2):341-362

[33] Collis E, Gavin J, Russell A, Brosnan M. Autistic adults' experience of restricted repetitive behaviours. Research in Autism Spectrum Disorders. 2022;**90**:101895

[34] Yu Y, Chaulagain A, Pedersen SA, Lydersen S, Leventhal BL, Szatmari P, et al. Pharmacotherapy of restricted/ repetitive behavior in autism spectrum disorder: A systematic review and meta-analysis. BMC Psychiatry. 2020;**20**(1):121

[35] Kinsbourne M. Repetitive movements and arousal. In: Fein DA, editor. The Neuropsychology of Autism. New York: Oxford University Press; 2011

[36] Lung SLM, Picard È, Soulières I, Bertone A. Identifying the functions of restricted and repetitive behaviours and interests in autism: A scoping review. Research in Autism Spectrum Disorders. 2024;**117**:102458

[37] McCormack L, Wong SW, Campbell LE. 'If I don't do it, I'm out of rhythm and I can't focus As well': Positive and negative adult interpretations of therapies aimed at 'fixing' their restricted and repetitive behaviours in childhood. Journal of Autism and Developmental Disorders. 2023;**53**(9):3435-3448

[38] Ekblad L, Pfuhl G. Autistic self-stimulatory behaviors (stims): Useless repetitive behaviors or nonverbal communication? Preprint on PsyArXiv. 18 Dec 2017. DOI: 10.31234/osf.io/4xyc2

[39] Kapp SK, Steward R, Crane L, Elliott D, Elphick C, Pellicano E, et al. 'People should be allowed to do what they like': Autistic adults' views and experiences of stimming. Autism. 2019;**23**(7):1782-1792

[40] Ekblad L. Autism, personality, and human diversity: Defining neurodiversity in an iterative process using aspie quiz. SAGE Open. 2013;**3**(3):2158244013497722

[41] Griffin E, Pollak D. Student experiences of neurodiversity in higher education: Insights from the BRAINHE Project. Dyslexia. 2009;**15**(1):23-41

[42] Jaarsma P, Welin S. Autism as a natural human variation: Reflections on the claims of the neurodiversity movement. Health Care Analysis. 2012;**20**(1):20-30

[43] Murray D, Milton D, Green J, Bervoets J. The human spectrum: A phenomenological enquiry within neurodiversity. Psychopathology. 2023;**56**(3):220-230

[44] World Medical Association Declaration of Helsinki. Ethical principles for medical research involving human subjects. Journal of

the American Medical Association. 2013;**310**(20):2191-2194

[45] R Development Core Team. R: A Language and Environment for Statistical Computing. Vienna, Austria: R Foundation for Statistical Computing; 2023

[46] JASP Team. JASP (Version 0.12.2) [Computer software]. 2020

[47] Diamond A. Executive functions. Annual Review of Psychology. 2013;**64**(1):135-168

[48] Ryan RM, Deci EL. Self-determination theory and the facilitation of intrinsic motivation, social development, and well-being. American Psychologist. 2000;**55**(1):68-78

[49] Murray AL, Booth T, McKenzie K, Kuenssberg R, O'Donnell M. Are autistic traits measured equivalently in individuals with and without an autism spectrum disorder? An invariance analysis of the autism spectrum quotient short form. Journal of Autism and Developmental Disorders. 2014;**44**(1):55-64

[50] Goldman S, Wang C, Salgado MW, Greene PE, Kim M, Rapin I. Motor stereotypies in children with autism and other developmental disorders. Developmental Medicine and Child Neurology. 2009;**51**(1):30-38

Chapter 7

# The Autistic Space Conjecture: Text/Field and the Individuals of Consciousness

*Noury Bakrim*


## Abstract

In this chapter, we expose an autistic space conjecture addressing a knowledge space of autism and its evaluation. The Real-Object-Approach of Language (ROAL)-hypothesis relies on an epistemic-mathematical model of autism adopting a framing/antiframing approach to linguistic/non-linguistic individuation of text/field varying from the pathological account on autism. The focus of the first phase is on the spectral plane of knowledge particles (linguistic/non-linguistic) by means of a parametric formula implying an autistic inversion of exponentiation of acts/facts and perception/production (representation) on the invariants of Action Cognition Emotion (CEA) taken as the individuals of consciousness and their exponents of Source-effectuator-target: it pinpoints spectral variation on perceptual spheres (intero/proprio/extero) whereby the framing/antiframing model yields a diathetic split proper to autism. The empirical/experimental verifiability of CEA individuals in autism relies particularly on random constructions and their differential search patterns. Within a monistic world, text/field configuration invariants indicate a mental space inwardly inverted on an Einsteinian/Galilean world. Thus, the first phase of the present work entails an applicability in which brain interconnectivity is considered, in particular hippocampal-cortical interactions. In sum, we proved a feasible method of *knowledge particles* on the autistic plane and its metrics of linguistic/non-linguistic individuals between individuation/configuration and individuality.


**Keywords:** antiframing, spectral plane, configuration, individuation, CEA individuals

## 1. Introduction

### 1.1 Introduction: The epistemic-mathematical frame and its modeling for language/impairment (autism)

The ROAL-Hypothesis has been conceived through different research and reflection phases, whose results could be read and checked from the following references [1–5]. It advocates a varying perspective on mathematical linguistics, from a bio-socio-mathematical framework in which cognome/connectome [6] and space considerations are stable components of neuro-verifiability, thanks to a monistic model of language stating that internalism/externalism can be rethought and reread by a bidirectional One-Text-Object (OTO) on sourcehood/acthood/targethood coordinates. Thus, by epistemic-mathematical frame, we do not mean applied Mathematical Linguistics (say, for instance, computational linguistics), nor do we mean by this term a new attempt on logical pragmatics.

By epistemic mathematics we do mean the mathematical foundation of the twofold text knowledge model: the knowing-epi / knowable-meta from first:

- Set-type-category interactions by means of typing *descending* operations (evaluations of universal verifiability) on the following axes endowed with semantic duality: syntax-discontinuous form, uttering-continuous form, rhythm, symmetry copying and categorical *ascending* objectification such as schematized by **Figure 1**.

On a manifold language reasoning with formula to allow calculus and algebra on linear/complex aspects of $epi^{meta}$ and reciprocal bijective functions (with natural language inductions). Our manifold model stipulates that the monistic language (Euclidean/non-Euclidean) space is a totally differentiable, linear/non-linear space whereby the entanglement states of observability/objectivity and associative axes on ${M^{fact}}_{act}$ (sourcehood, acthood, targethood) are represented by way of manifold mapping $R^n \rightarrow R^{2n} \rightarrow R^3(R^2)$ considering X, Y, Z arguments, we distinguish verifiability from surface bivariate selection on $R^3$ on the physical space of observation. We, secondly, consider one arrow directionality of Source-Effectuator-Target and event of lambda-individuation (lambda individual language operations) on random occurrences, we also define a solvability notion of parameters.

Nonetheless, the duality theorem of the ROAL, especially on neurodiverse conjecture, stipulates an Autistic Language Space that entails spectrum condition being a knowing plane. We, thus, hypothesize the following outline in **Figure 2**.

### 1.2 The framing/antiframing duality and its measurement

Independently from Jakobson-Kurt approach of language pathology [7], where both symbolic and instrumental are the core hypothesis of pathological causality on language, the above-outlined model aims at addressing the dual framing of autism from spectrum relevance. Henceforth, the framing/antiframing duality is the duality in which we can read the language knowledge space of autism. Polarity and spectral dimensions will be described and defined later.

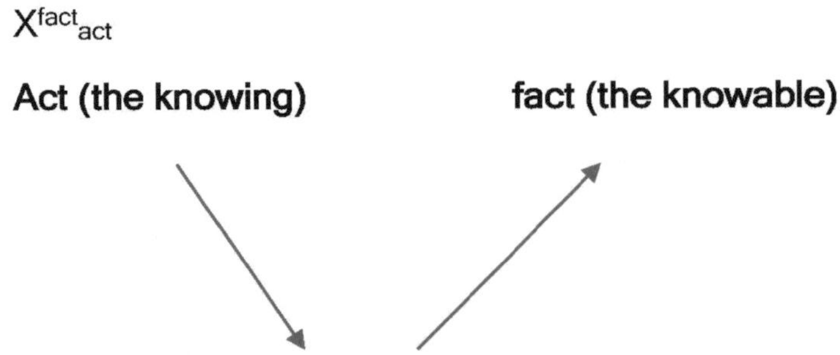


**Figure 1.**
*The trivial space of text bidirectionality.*

*DOI: http://dx.doi.org/10.5772/intechopen.1010189*

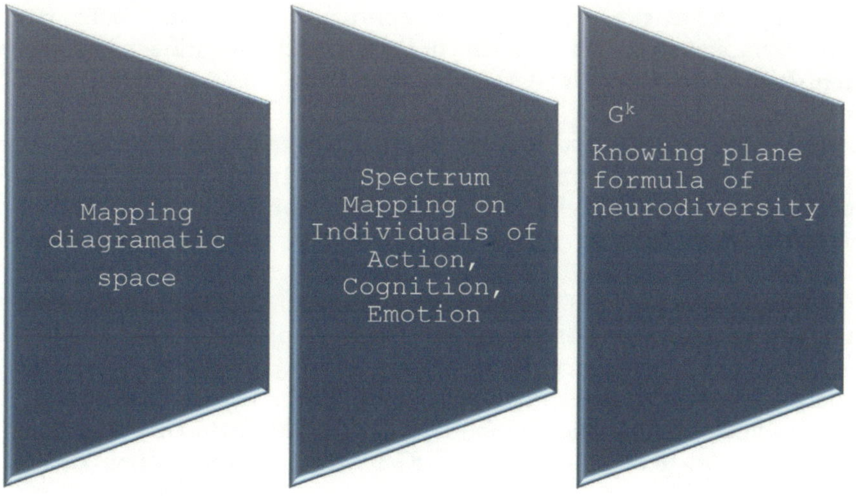


**Figure 2.**
*Spectrum condition plane.*

### *1.2.1 The proper epistemic manifold of autism (from 2021-hypothesis)*

The following element has been conjectured in the following observation: *"Why can a 4-years autistic child build a complex puzzle of 150 pieces with complex notions of science fiction in less than five minutes (a space station with its control tower and complex architectural accessories including a multicolor decorum)?* To reduce it to a mathematical hypothetic dealing, we adopt the following markers: let us consider the space X on the two-dimensional surface $S^2$ being the surface of the puzzle whose flat Euclidean set containing the collection of inclusive subsets formed by the pieces $\{p_1, \ldots p_n\}$ such that each piece is seen by the non-autistic child as subsets p, $p \subset Sf$ or the set of the flat surface and the space X' seen by the autistic child being a topological space with the collection of hyperbolic curve surfaces that are diffeomorphic to each other forming the collection of the set of boundary sets $B_{set}$ with metric space considerations. Therefore, returning to Riemann tensor, the autistic child does not see the difference between flat and curved derivation while the non-autistic child must perform the tensor relation. The puzzle result is inserted on the flat dimension that has been metrically converted to/from the Euclidean setting while the hyperbolic perspective sees connections of geodesic levels" [8].

The choice of a *non-linguistic observed* (to discern it from *observable*) points out toward a particularly important methodological nuance, the double structuring of linguistic/extra-linguistic structures. It has its relevance in the ternary structure of the Real (sourcehood, acthood, targethood) along with its individual output (Action, Cognition, Emotion), at the core element of argument structure within the monistic manifolding. Retaking the same observational conjecture, the double structuring has a different mental/physical "exposition scene" within manifolding, regardless of the classifying mathematical dimension on manifold objects between nature and culture.

The mapping dynamic as a space transformation pinpoints a different relation between surface, plane and projections. From the ontic individuation principle, geometrical typology principle (surface/hypersurface, parameters, equations ... ) can be approached by the principle of *configuration.* Before referring to theoretical sources of configuration principle, we ground in Gestalt, especially *Modular Manifoldness* [9].

- *Tensegrity*: The tension and integrity of configuration on individuated structures [10–12] implies a relation between continuous and discontinuous members (tensiles/links and strats/nodes).
- *Driesch vitalism and entelechy*: From Hydra equipotential distribution, where the whole as a footprint is expressed in parts: Especially, addressing field situatedness in morphogenesis of the embryo cell with its upper and lower gradients (valence encoding) [13, 14].
- *The Bühlerian feld/field*: Bühler language theory underpinned with psychological foundations points out Gestalt principles of the inner and the surrounding field, it can be read off the distinctions of the organon-model; utterly designating the deictic (Zeigefeld), representational (Darstellungsfeld or metalinguistic dimensions) and symbolic (Symbolfeld) levels. This is the first attempt on *dynamic totality* to text/field (inner and surrounding) and configuration of wholes [9, 15].

Thus, to bring these elements to a coherent inquiry, we introduce the following axiomatic statement:

> *Dynamic totality in autism relies on maps of differential categories along with diffeomorphic or the differential structure that vary along gradients of individuated and field configuration as shown by* **Table 1**.

We redefine this duality within a diathesis expression from bidirectionality to CEA individuals whereby text/field formulas obtain a specification relating to their polarity. Therefore, one can state that exponentiation changes following diathesis polarity. Thus, we propose the following expressions:

- Participational event diathesis: $act_{p1}{}^{fact\ p1}/\ fact_{p2}{}^{act\ p2}$
- Act event diathesis (action/emotion): $A^E$ / $E^A$
- Neurotype event diathesis: $K^g/G^k$

Equipped with these terms, we emphasize a second declension relating to the proper perceptual space of autism (its imbalance in the etiology/pathology of the phenomenon), especially the interaction between three perceptual spheres, interoceptive, proprioceptive and exteroceptive domains [16–18]. We should nonetheless stress that these considerations have been reread from the monistic framework. Henceforth, beyond the autistic act polarity, we reconsider three gradients from G that represent the three spheres: $G_{int}$, $G_{prop}$ and $G_{exter}$ enable us to describe the interactions between them in a mode in which they, hypothetically and internally,

| Frame: $K^g$ | Antiframe: $G^k$ |
|---|---|
| • Text/field stable field configuration of surfaces (linear/non-linear/flat-curved) | • Text/field varying configuration of surface/plane relations |

**Table 1.**
*Framing duality.*

redefine another dimension of the CEA individuals, especially the applicability of their invariant exponents (source, effectuator, target). As per the physical dimension of sensory percepts, particle/wave modeling relation between seeing/hearing (wave/particle-like) and touching, smelling, tasting (non-wave) opens a relation between wave (photon/phonon) and non-wave modeling, which advocates for representational exponentiation (also by semantic dualities) where we also reintroduce the Lotmanian idea of first and secondary modeling systems in language [19]. In this sense, the dualistic frame (from dualism, to be distinguished from logical dualities) will be replaced by our monistic representational approach.

Moreover, reintroducing the configuration debate, the interplay of text/field structure and the random individuation is somehow "mediated" by the parametric value of $G^k$ in respect of $epi^{meta}$ knowledge representation whereby we hypothesize a second applicability of the procedural knowledge on autistic perceptual spheres of intero-proprio-exteroceptive domains (perceptual autistic *acts* from exponent parameters with potential of *vicarious perception* [20]). Therefore, a split in neurotype could be postulated between:

- Structure / individuation or the process of tensegrity that reconsiders the knowledge formula into an *individual structure* (with random configuration/ random mapping).

- Individuality / individuation or the very autistic process of doubled randomness of Hebbian apperceptive processes [21, 22] regarding brain/real-world assemblies.

#### *1.2.2 The new hypothesis: $G^k$ knowing plane of autism*

The relation between manifold and its configuration, mediated by mathematical topology classification (differentiable manifolds, compactness, connectedness, cobordism), suggests an epistemic space of language, especially the existence of polyhedral properties [9] under simplicial triangulation and the constructs of simplicial classification. Thus, the hull formed by simplicial hyperbolic curves from vertices on P and polytope conditions of convex/concave pushing/pulling on surfaces and hypersurfaces (in particular, flat/curved considerations) may be regarded from Action/ Cognition/Emotion individuals and their linguistic/non-linguistic common invariants.

- *The fixed coordinate/associative frame of text/field*:

Sourcehood/Acthood/Targethood as designed by **Figure 3** (fixed coordinates).

- *The neurotypical framing: linguistic/non-linguistic model of CEA exposition along with rotational qualia such as summed up by* **Figure 4**.

Sourcehood-Acthood-Targethood (source-effectuator-target).

xzx, yzy, zyz, xyz, xyx, zxz / source-target-source, effectuator-source-effectuator, target-effectuator-target, source-effectuator-source, target-source-target following the model of **Figure 5**.

considering rotational angle framing in which the linguistic component of the Real (field) on CEA is the schematized event (ontic qualia) on exponents from verb argument applicability such that Action (motor-oriented), Emotion (sensory-

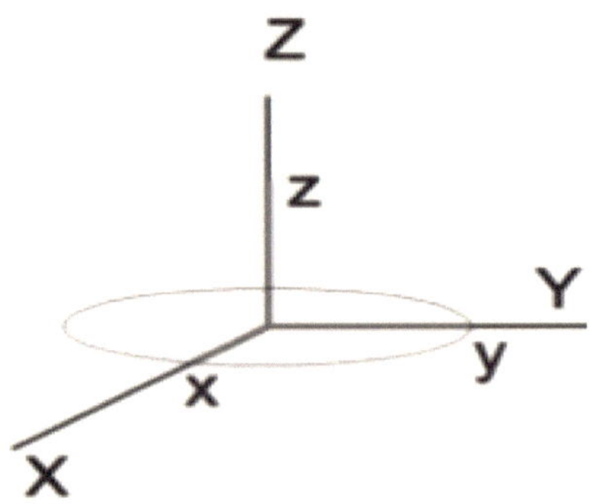


**Figure 3.**
*Fixed coordinates.*

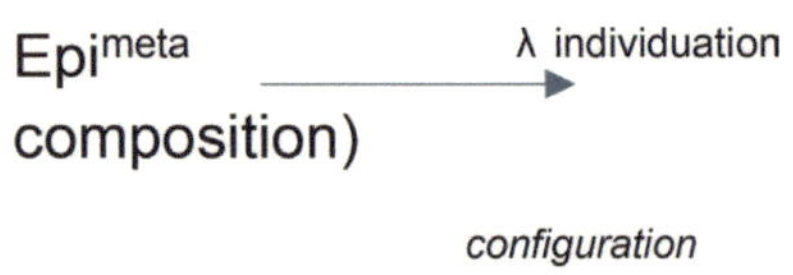


**Figure 4.**
*Individuation and composition.*

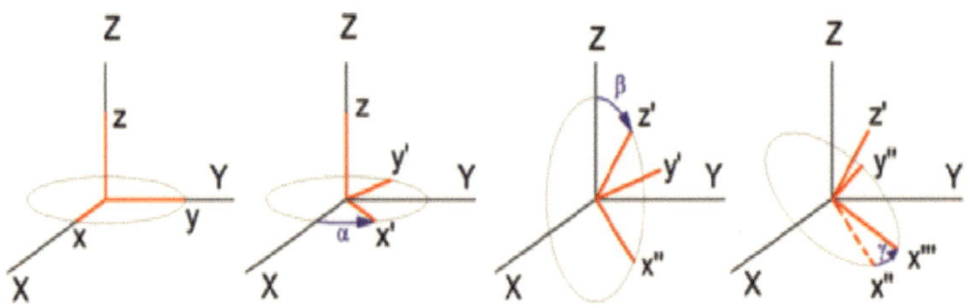


**Figure 5.**
*Fixed/rotating angles.*

oriented) and Cognition (Representation with semantic and notional exponentiation) apply source-effectuator-target (discrete random) on frames (acquisition of combinatorial symmetry on syntax-driven semantic representation within anthropolinguistic field experience), situation (morpho-dynamic uttering events) and expositions (morpho-discontinuous events from valence and verb classes).

- *The antiframing or the autistic knowing plane*

Following the sense given by our abovementioned conjecture, tensegrity, being an abstract principle of configured individuals (non-applied, non-technical at this stage), implies hypersurface dealing from text individuation along with the description of individuation. The canonical formula $G^k$ with cross-descriptive parameters will be applied to variant-invariant antiframing considerations. It also suggests the probability of building random walks on the configuration of the Real with computing consequences and input/output directions on both linguistic/non-linguistic in the following sense given by individuation → configuration (tensegrity) → output. The gradient can be broken down into various aspects of the spectrum.

*DOI: http://dx.doi.org/10.5772/intechopen.1010189*

- *Entropy/prime number in autistic antiframing*

The spectrum exerts a constraint on entropy computation by prime numbers with specific focus on antiframed distribution of entropy by prime numbers. In this regard, we hypothesize prime number gap applicability to be bearing on N-recruited population of neurons (also under the neurodegenerative consideration) and N-number of individuals modeling the symptomatic "observed" on one side, and between individuals on the other side. Inversely, number theoretical considerations are to be ascribed to the debate on hippocampus-cortex interactions (or number specificity from category-set relations) where number object from categories, especially natural number objects, can be induced in algebraic set frame [23].

We, thus, adopting covariance of prime numbers between (neuron, individuals/individual-individual) aspects aim at constructing modular deficit on distribution in the spectral antiframing. Furthermore, from plane consideration, restarting/resuming dimensions on exponent's rotation yields another significance when dealing with observation of repetitive behavior, echolalia, truncation (from our non-pathological accounts) ... .in particular, the spiral side of multiple zeros on zeta-analytic function grounding in **Figure 6** [24].

*1.2.3 Individuals and symptomatic measurement: The spectrum*

One of the major challenges of the present section is the symptomatic description and measurement of linguistic/non-linguistic CEA individuals. Therefore, we focus on field parameters pinpointing relevant access to this purpose. The invariant modeling of the symptoms points out toward Infeld/Umfeld (inner/surrounding field interactions). Moreover, considering the spectrum within antiframing, we postulate from matrix linearity, transition states (stochastic) on event/occurrence starting from the smallest entropy measure generated by prime number gaps [25]. Secondly, under linear/complex parts, entropy variation seems to be a random spectral path on the observation setting. In addition, applicability of symptoms (from individuation) requires a first mapping attempt. Before any further dealing, we emphasize that variation itself is mapped through an empirical mathematical process of domain coloring.

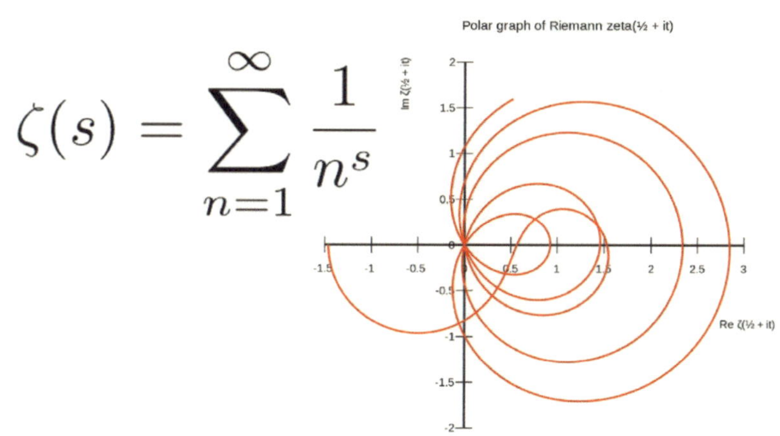


**Figure 6.**
*Multiple zeros on zeta analytic function.*

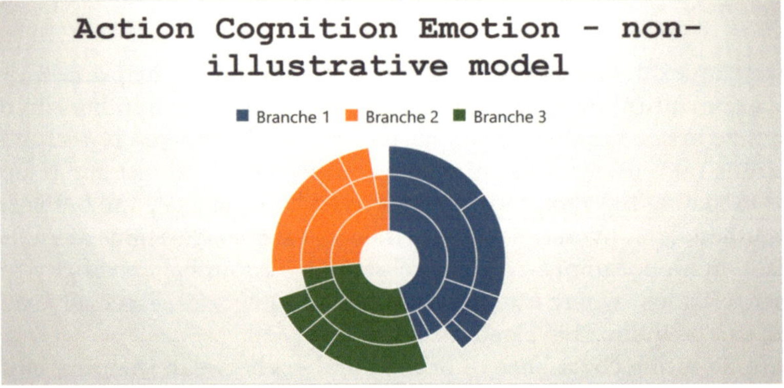


**Figure 7.**
*The non-illustrative model.*

| Individuals | | Observation | | | | |
|---|---|---|---|---|---|---|
| | | Symptomatic input | | Observable output | | directionality |
| Action Cognition Emotion | Action linguistic exponents | **Observed** | **Knowing field** | **Field/text relevant level** | **Exponent applicable** | $G^K$ |
| | | e.g truncation | Infeld/Umfeld (neurodiverse) | Verb valence 'donner glace' | Source → target | |
| | **Action non-linguistic exponents** | e.g motion toward the fridge | Umfeld / Infeld (neurotypical) | Motion | effectuator→ target | $K^g$ |

**Table 2.**
*Invariant.*

Hence, from spectrum result representation, empirical conditions redefine a synthetic knowing plane whereby a symptomatic plotting varies within other parameters. However, reinterpreting this element enables the representation of invariant observables within a non-illustrative model of magnitude (appearing from the plane of observation through the spectrum of **Figure** 7).

Taking the invariants to be symptomatically observed from framing/antiframing variation, we define a first common in **Table 2.**

The applied module will be defined by the experimental setting (invariant / variant). In addition, the observation principle relies on a sequencing model implying multiple embedding of individuals and their exponents within the frame. Therefore, semiotic duality arises from the proper scientific field of the object.

- *Semiotic duality from object field*:

From our semiotic duality model [26], we stipulate a lower dimension for semiotics in **Figure** 8. However, grounding in the sequencing predicate principle obtained from multiple embedding, CEA individuals are defined, thanks to integration of linguistic/non-linguistic invariants in which a second distinction becomes necessary in **Figure** 9.

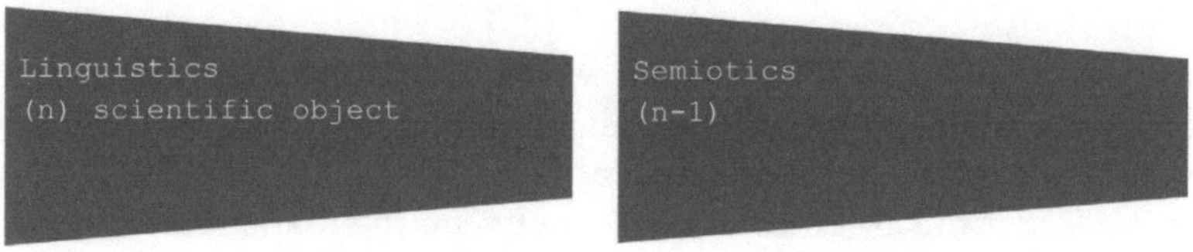


**Figure 8.**
*Semiotic duality.*

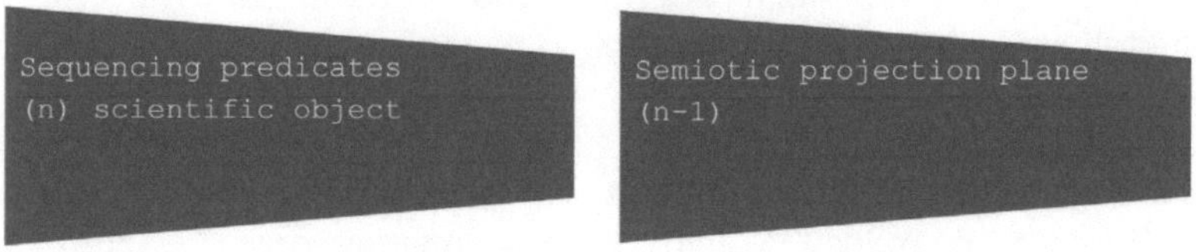


**Figure 9.**
*Semiotic Projection Plane.*

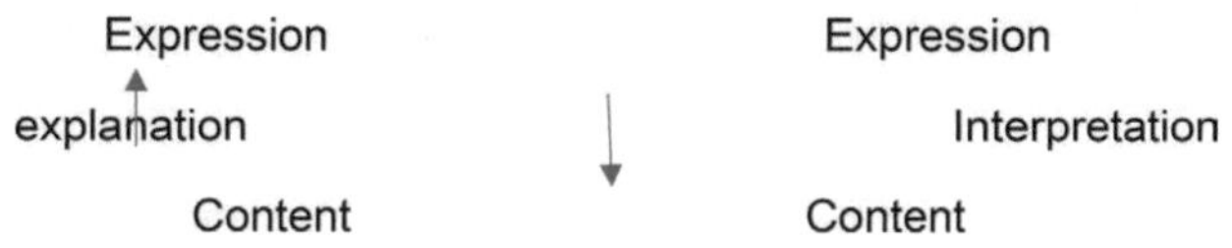


**Figure 10.**
*Explanation/interpretation.*

The semiotic plane, unlike the mythological-fictional frame of French semiotics [27], is a measuring observation tool where we generate different methodological levels such as explanation and interpretation. Direction of the observation is provided by the projective line model from the polarity of the duality such as demonstrated by **Figure 10**.

In which case, symptomatic variables are shaped by sequencing propositions and their field interpretants along spectrum gradients of diversity.

## 2. Individuals within a monistic brain-consciousness

The monistic brain-consciousness, part of the ROAL-model, aims at understanding and explaining field monism and its implication on language-individual language phenomena. Field implications within brain connectome-cognome (cortical networks) ground in interconnectivity [28–30]. From brain entropy, especially from entanglement states of observability and objectivity, the in-out states replace deductive principles of inference. Furthermore, event-related potential (ERP) probability, whereby a Bayesian scheme and other related non-deterministic aspects can be conceived, has some consequences on the present assumptions. Among those, the shift into a graph theoretical frame without losing viewpoint on the knowing plane. This very spatialization by graph models entails that connectome-cognome interactions are regarded as a frame of field individuals where a monadic heuristic can be conceived; modularity of random graphs within brain-consciousness may then be viewed as access to the self-expansion/self-reduction proposal spaces [31]. Hence, functional interconnectivity from hemispheric applicability may be defined by the same observation of the knowing plane (its spectral model). Moreover, self-assembly dimensions of the field previously posited and discussed [26] orientate the abovementioned debate toward a monistic invariant frame where, beyond synchronization states, the question of the manifold, especially mapping translation on the three-dimensional (3D) physical space, has been raising recent neurological debates [32].

Yet, we think that the absent distinction between the mathematical-epistemic significance of $R^3$ and lower-dimensional manifold (without the typological approach on topological objects) misses the relation between conscious spaces within an Einsteinian-Galilean world mathematically modeled. In this regard, the debate on the connectome, where we distinguish functional and neural-graph connectome [33], includes the following hypothetic elements.

- The differential conjecture of autism [34]: non-differential manifolds (no vector space to allow algebra) do not depend on a differentiation structure Dm endowed with diffeomorphic maps [35] $Dm_1 \rightarrow Dm_2$, in which case spectrum variation metric will have to include differential variation parameters, especially from the following model between abstract manifolding and its 3-Manifold properties (cortex). Therefore, this differentiability is given by a graph-spatialization (implicitly, discretely defined) from a decomposition nature, potentially, through both transition maps and $R^3$ translation.

An overview on abstract mathematical properties of the manifold on $R^n/C^n$ is given by **Figure 11**.

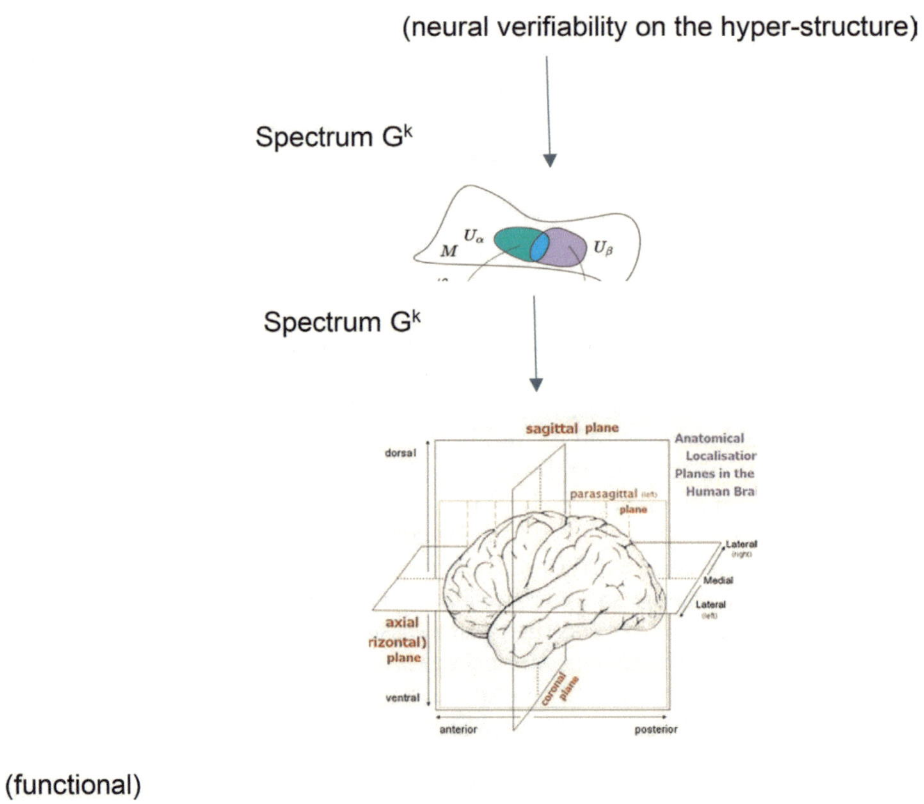


**Figure 11.**
*Brain manifold.*

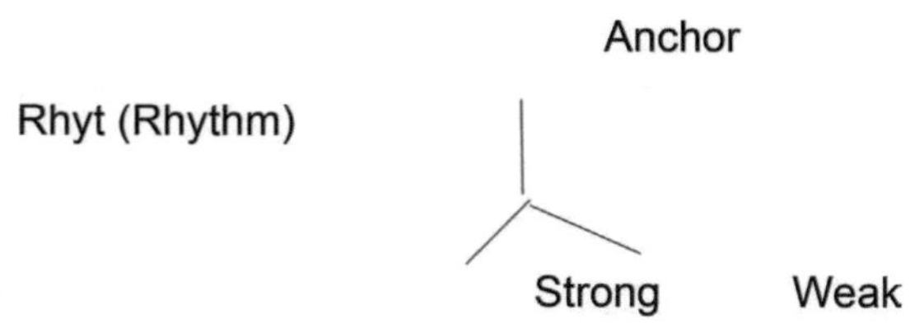


**Figure 12.**
*In – out graphs of truth-conditional verifiability on epistemic neural, parallel-antiparallel graphs.*

Another scheme is the category-set decomposition of manifolds into cell-like sets whereby a neighborhood of points can be contracted to a U point [36]. In this case, Hippocampus-Cortex interactions need to be reconsidered.

### 2.1 Dynome imbalance

Excitatory/inhibitory imbalance [37, 38] is regarded in our epistemic frame as a spectral variation on hyper-hyposensitivity and therefore relating higher abstract to lower abstract connectome predicates. Thus, the correlates of the lower dimension of cortex, in terms of connectomic neurotypicality, are regarded as varying currying/uncurrying patterns of rhythmic universal graph of verifiability by means of varying partition patterns (**Figure 12**) *on epistemic neural, parallel-antiparallel graphs*.

### 2.2 Category-set symmetrical brain in $G^k$

Group and category transformation, especially in group symmetry, is a group action on sets enabling mapping and cycle generation. In this sense, from Mirror Neuron System (MNS) [39, 40] and its link to language properties (our text level of acquisition axis) we consider a conjecture on symmetric mapping in the sense of group generation on cortex functional connectome of learning regarding CEA individuals.

The purpose of learnability from the model of deep and surface layers has been reinterpreting ontogenetic and epigenetic modification of Mirror Neurons (mother-child social experience). The graph reinterpreting model [41] addressing the insertion of dominating set properties from Gr1 to Gr2 (mother / Child) suggests additivity of premotor Mirror System in Gr3 (learning graph). Hence, we hypothesize a categorification through enrichment for learnability [42, 43], especially symmetric maps and enriched sets that meet matching biological properties [44] of replisome and connectome at the intersection of a spectral variation on category (hippocampal neurons) and sets (cognomic/connectomic graphs).

Set group generators are defined as symmetric categories and their enriched set categories $Set_{cat}$ of both learnability and coupling purposes (enabling object from binary couples for instance) on one object (monoidal category). Therefore, enrichment of XYZ implies an internal unifying object with symmetry and tensoring properties allowing for combinatorial and vector sets. Diagrammatic enrichment variation on the knowing plane is hypothesized, put in relation to coupling operations of symmetry and learnability.

## 3. Testing the autistic space conjecture: The first phase

In the following attempt, we trace the contours of conjecture's applicability and feasibility, by evaluating its specificity as a knowing space, instead of a pathological/

therapeutic approach on the latter. Therefore, we present here an experimental setting relying on a mathematical-epistemic method (first phase of the experiment).

### 3.1 The procedure

In the present ongoing research, we met the parents of medically diagnosed children with Autism Spectrum Disorder (ASD) condition within the hosting frame of the SOS Autisme Casablanca, which is one of the leading associations in educational-social care in Morocco (website). Secondly, we submitted an agreement consisting of juridical acceptance from parent/legal representative sides and declining extra/intra-academic conflicts of interest. A questionnaire aiming at knowing the autistic children from the perspective of age, gender, spectrum condition and speaking/non-speaking status, comorbidity and risk factors has been given to the parents and legal representatives. It is made up of three components: A, B, C standing for data comparison (between observation and diagnosis data) and personal data on linguistic/non-linguistic individuals of CEA. The questionnaire has been designed in French to match educational background of Moroccan caregivers, doctors and parents, even if the semi-directive has been conducted in Moroccan Darija for more convenience and easier data collection. The aim was to collect earlier data for field and interaction observation. As such, it is not meant to be used in a proposal on diagnosis.

We observed, in a second phase, linguistic and non-linguistic interactions within physical space. Videos and photos of the participants with caregivers, together and alone, enable a second basis for the present conjecture.

### 3.2 Method and results

Given a declension principle of the knowing space conjecture consisting of the integration of the framing/antiframing hypothesis into a mapping method along with its metric on both scalar/vector fields [45], we relied, first, on the bidirectional real/complex formula from $\text{epi}^{\text{meta}}$ XYZ coordinates elements. To reconsider individuals' invariants and exponents on linguistic/non-linguistic, we applied a non-pathological/non-therapeutic definition of the knowing space to specify the meta-aspect within the conditions of rotation and motion that are necessary to individuation and their bivariate random representation of the field (the field of the Real). Thus, mapping autistic spectrum on a plane implies Euler Angle Matrices on rotation, of which intrinsic (rotation angles on the fixed XYZ frame) and extrinsic (rotation angles on the reference frame), following both models of Euler (left) and Tait (right) [46] or **Table 3** model.

It allows us to introduce a first representation of knowing plane linearity. On the other hand, we adopt a complex gradient operator [45], being direction of the scalar field (from surface observation) and derivability/variation of the complex side of the analytic function. In this regard, optimizing this gradient on the complex/real knowing plane is also defining it in its particular case "a vector operator which gives the direction of the steepest ascent of a real-scalar valued function" [47]. A holomorphic function (real/complex) duality of integration/differentiation is secondly considered.

Given the latter, z = a complex variable,

$$z = x + jy \tag{1}$$

with a real valued function, given a non-linear functional $df_c$ (.) on the tangent space $C_z{}^n$

*DOI: http://dx.doi.org/10.5772/intechopen.1010189*

| | |
|---|---|
| $Y_\alpha X_\beta Y_\gamma = \begin{bmatrix} c_\alpha c_\gamma - c_\beta s_\alpha s_\gamma & s_\alpha s_\beta & c_\alpha s_\gamma + c_\beta c_\gamma s_\alpha \\ s_\beta s_\gamma & c_\beta & -c_\gamma s_\beta \\ -c_\gamma s_\alpha - c_\alpha c_\beta s_\gamma & c_\alpha s_\beta & c_\alpha c_\beta c_\gamma - s_\alpha s_\gamma \end{bmatrix}$ | $Y_\alpha X_\beta Z_\gamma = \begin{bmatrix} c_\alpha c_\gamma + s_\alpha s_\beta s_\gamma & c_\gamma s_\alpha s_\beta - c_\alpha s_\gamma & c_\beta s_\alpha \\ c_\beta s_\gamma & c_\beta c_\gamma & -s_\beta \\ c_\alpha s_\beta s_\gamma - c_\gamma s_\alpha & c_\alpha c_\gamma s_\beta + s_\alpha s_\gamma & c_\alpha c_\beta \end{bmatrix}$ |
| $Y_\alpha Z_\beta Y_\gamma = \begin{bmatrix} c_\alpha c_\beta c_\gamma - s_\alpha s_\gamma & -c_\alpha s_\beta & c_\gamma s_\alpha + c_\alpha c_\beta s_\gamma \\ c_\gamma s_\beta & c_\beta & s_\beta s_\gamma \\ -c_\alpha s_\gamma - c_\beta c_\gamma s_\alpha & s_\alpha s_\beta & c_\alpha c_\gamma - c_\beta s_\alpha s_\gamma \end{bmatrix}$ | $Y_\alpha Z_\beta X_\gamma = \begin{bmatrix} c_\alpha c_\beta & s_\alpha s_\gamma - c_\alpha c_\gamma s_\beta & c_\gamma s_\alpha + c_\alpha s_\beta s_\gamma \\ s_\beta & c_\beta c_\gamma & -c_\beta s_\gamma \\ -c_\beta s_\alpha & c_\alpha s_\gamma + c_\gamma s_\alpha s_\beta & c_\alpha c_\gamma - s_\alpha s_\beta s_\gamma \end{bmatrix}$ |
| $Z_\alpha Y_\beta Z_\gamma = \begin{bmatrix} c_\alpha c_\beta c_\gamma - s_\alpha s_\gamma & -c_\gamma s_\alpha - c_\alpha c_\beta s_\gamma & c_\alpha s_\beta \\ c_\alpha s_\gamma + c_\beta c_\gamma s_\alpha & c_\alpha c_\gamma - c_\beta s_\alpha s_\gamma & s_\alpha s_\beta \\ -c_\gamma s_\beta & s_\beta s_\gamma & c_\beta \end{bmatrix}$ | $Z_\alpha Y_\beta X_\gamma = \begin{bmatrix} c_\alpha c_\beta & c_\alpha s_\beta s_\gamma - c_\gamma s_\alpha & s_\alpha s_\gamma + c_\alpha c_\gamma s_\beta \\ c_\beta s_\alpha & c_\alpha c_\gamma + s_\alpha s_\beta s_\gamma & c_\gamma s_\alpha s_\beta - c_\alpha s_\gamma \\ -s_\beta & c_\beta s_\gamma & c_\beta c_\gamma \end{bmatrix}$ |
| $\begin{bmatrix} c_\alpha c_\gamma - c_\beta s_\alpha s_\gamma & -c_\alpha s_\gamma - c_\beta c_\gamma s_\alpha & s_\alpha s_\beta \end{bmatrix}$ | $\begin{bmatrix} c_\alpha c_\gamma - s_\alpha s_\beta s_\gamma & -c_\beta s_\alpha & c_\alpha s_\gamma + c_\gamma s_\alpha s_\beta \end{bmatrix}$ |

**Table 3.**
*Euler/Tait angles.*

$$\mathrm{Df_c(v)} = 2\ \mathrm{Re}\left\{\frac{\partial f(c)}{\partial z}.v\right\} \tag{2}$$

$$\mathrm{V} \in \mathrm{C_z}^{\mathrm{n}}\ \mathrm{c} = (\mathrm{z}, z^{-})$$

Henceforth, gradient/gradient operator formula can be written, thanks to the following operations

- Gradient of, $f$ (knowing space function) [45]

$$\nabla_z f \triangleq \Omega_z^{-1}\left(\frac{\partial f}{\partial z}\right)^{\mathrm{H}} \tag{3}$$

$$\nabla_{\mathrm{z}}(.) \triangleq \Omega_z^{-1}\left(\frac{\partial(.)}{\partial z}\right)^{\mathrm{H}} \tag{4}$$

We then consider this operator as g, a diversity gradient of the autistic space. Inversely, the trace of rotation matrices (or the traces of the knowing space) k is written as the sum additivity trace of its eigenvalues on $(nxn)$ matrices or

$$\mathrm{Tr}\ (\mathrm{A}) = \sum\nolimits_{i=1}^{n} aii \tag{5}$$

$$= \mathrm{a}_{11} + \mathrm{a}_{22} + \ldots \mathrm{a}_{\mathrm{nn}}$$

Hence

$$\mathrm{K(t)} = \lambda_{\mathrm{intr}} + \lambda_{\mathrm{extrin}} \tag{6}$$

or the additivity of intrinsic and extrinsic rotation frames from the individuals' exponent of source-effectuator-target. We consider, therefore, the exponentiation

$$\mathrm{G}^{\mathrm{K}}\ \text{or}\ \mathrm{K_n} = \mathrm{G}^{\mathrm{k}} \tag{7}$$

metric (for which the neurotypical framing is the exponential inversion $\mathrm{K}^{\mathrm{g}}$).

The knowing plane obtention using complex exponentiation from G, complex gradient space (linearly independent vector basis) and k traces implies that z = x + iy when applied to the complex frame of exponentiation yields Euler constant relevance. Using Euler formulas will be a generating model from Euler solvability set

$$e^{x+iy} = e^{x} \cos\ y + ie^{x} \sin\ y \tag{8}$$

$$e^{i\pi} = \cos\ \pi + i\ \sin\ \pi \tag{9}$$

$$y = e^{x} \tag{10}$$

secondly, epistemization of g-gradient enables us to reinterpret $G^k$ from within the graph of complex exponentiation, in which case it will serve as a behavior of the latter in the following sense where polar coordinates can be conceived, y being the imaginary and x the real part shown by **Figure 13**.

To plot the multiple zero and entropy gaps: from the abovementioned considerations on entropy (less/more) and autistic spectrum, entropy distribution and variation will be optimized by the multiple zero aspects (see zeta function frame), especially for the right-hand side (critical non-trivial zeros).

Reinterpreting y and x from randomness frame. Shannon entropy

$$\text{H (k)} = \sum\nolimits_{i=1}^{n} P(ki)\, log\, 2P(ki) \tag{11}$$

$P(ki)$ is the probability mass function of the discrete random variables k (k1 ... kn).

The random walk generated by prime gaps:

On $Z^2$, we consider random walks on the surface of representation (mental/physical surface), stochastic transition matrices on k-matrices with epistemic basis set from k = trace of a matrix.

On a finite state space ith and jth row matrix probability

$$\text{P (j/i)} = P_{I/j} \tag{12}$$

and

$$\sum\nolimits_{j=1}^{\infty} Pij = 1 \tag{13}$$

And

$$\begin{bmatrix} T^{00} & \cdots & T^{0D} \\ \vdots & \ddots & \vdots \\ T^{D0} & \cdots & T^{DD} \end{bmatrix}$$

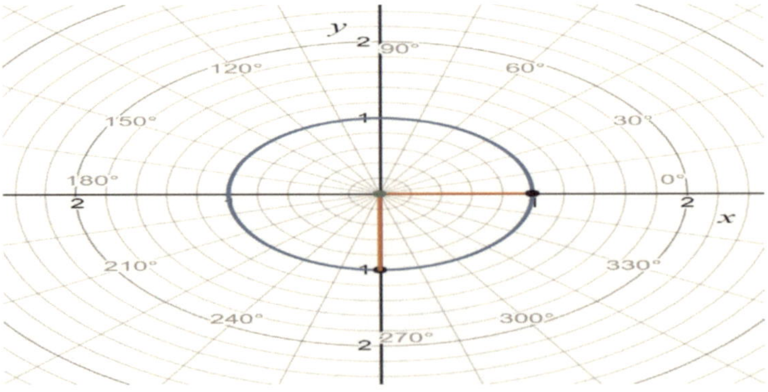


**Figure 13.**
*Spectral plane.*

Then on a finite state of random individuals, from rotation matrix frame we redefine the subsets of K and g through z discrete representation of a process designating zones of successful and failure sequences [48, 49] mapped by **Figure 14**.

### 3.3 Spectral plane and score representation

The principles of a spectral representation have been exposited in the abovementioned elements on the knowing space conjecture. Moreover, studies have shown circular plane relevance for random walk, especially particle probability states. We, herein, propose the following representation in a spectral plane from a concentric plane with center C and radius R1, radius R2, radius R3 [50–52] or **Figure 15**.

From Laplace solution equation, we obtain a probability for a knowable particle (we distinguish in the ROAL-model between particulate and participational arguments) to get absorbed at angle $\vartheta$.

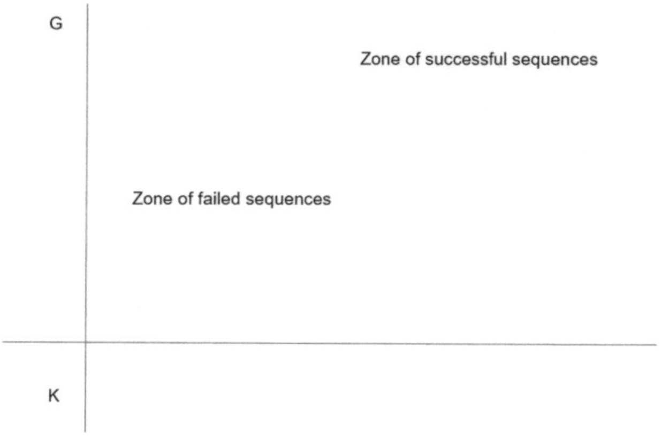


**Figure 14.**
*Sequence zones.*

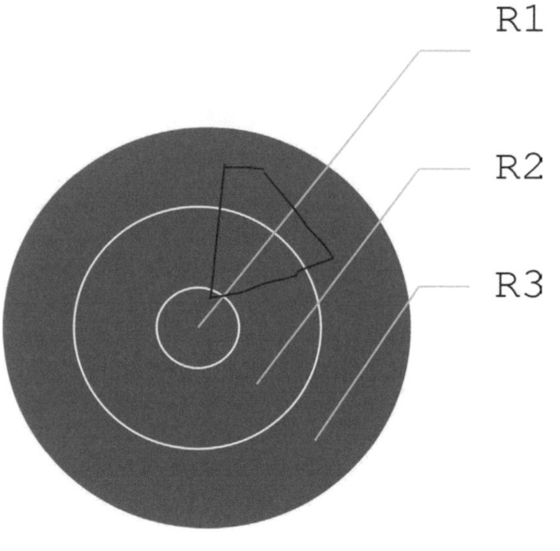


**Figure 15.**
*Score representation.*

$$P\ (\vartheta) = 1/2\varpi\ \left(x^2 - 1\right)/\left(x^2 - 2x\cos\ \vartheta + 1\right) \tag{14}$$

With respect to particle non-directional motion on the spectral plane, we apply randomness (discrete random variable on event individuation of CEA)

$$\Theta = f\ (v) = 2\ \arctan\ (x - 1/x + 1\tan\ v\ \varpi/2) \tag{15}$$

V being a random number,

$$v \in [-1, 1]\ \text{and}\ x = R2/R1\ 1 \tag{16}$$

Secondly, angles formed by epistemic particles can be described using epistemic exponents of source, effectuator, target. We propose the following mapping on the scoring measure of individuals which grounds in the $G^k$ frame, where G is a complex variable and k linear spectrum score scale with finite integers 1, 2, 3 … .

In so doing, we reconsider the randomness of CEA zones within the spectral (polar plane) from event results shaped by angle formation: first angles/randomness, then three zone formations of 120°. The experimental measuring process of epistemic particles can be conceived from the same considerations.

### *3.3.1 A differential model on stochastic considerations: The spectral search of boundary using Brownian motion*

The differential relevance of the present purpose relates to event random maps. In this sense, from our diffeomorphic hypothesis, a second differential stochastic equation can be applied to the epistemic process [53].

$$dX_t = \mu(Xt, t)dt + \sigma(Xt, t)dBt \tag{17}$$

whereby Brownian Motion is the constant B entailing patterns of variance and squared behavior of the epistemic patterns.

The second option will be the Gaussian noise

$$Dx\ (t)/dt = F\ (x(t)) + \sum\nolimits_{\alpha=1} g_\alpha(x(t))\zeta(t)^\alpha \tag{18}$$

The plotting simulacra of the process can be conceived for both individual and collective (independent random variables) "epistemic search," it takes its condition from the spectral complex plane. In a second endeavor, we define from the Brownian motion, the boundary space of points within the complex knowing plane (spectral plane). Thanks to a h-function on a complex plane [54], in **Figure 16** we plot $\partial k$ or the space of knowing/knowable autistic boundaries.

In so doing, we measure how the Brownian motion is distributed from a base point with a second property that computes the points on $\partial k$ since "planar Brownian Motion is recurrent but does not see points" [55]. Moreover, since we already have angle considerations in $k$-terms, we apply the harmonic function family along with Brownian Motion process already mapped. In this regard, $C^K$ endows the process with its points in the following sense,

Under conformal maps (preserving angles/angle probability), we obtain:

$$G^k\ \text{with}\ z_0 = 1 \tag{19}$$

With image/preimage from Brownian motion or **Figure 17.**

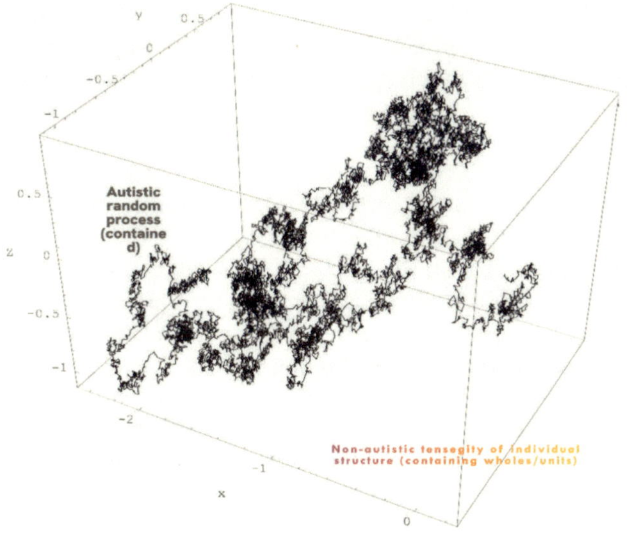


**Figure 16.**
*Autistic/non-autistic hypothesis of individuality-individuation.*

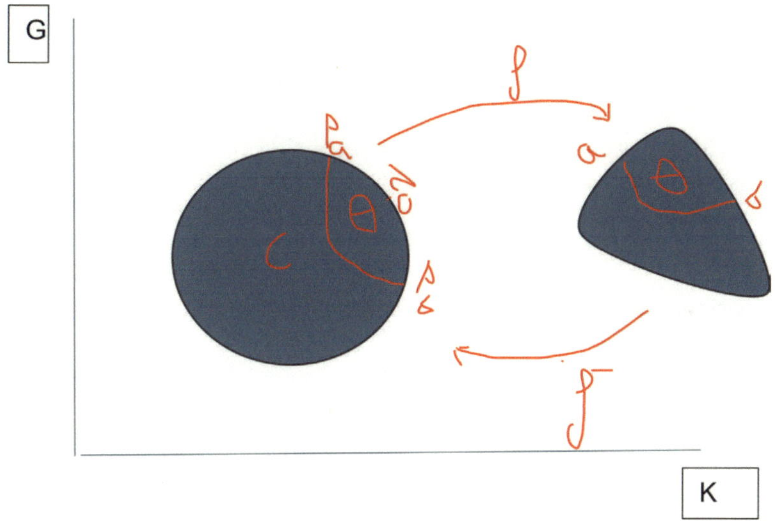


**Figure 17.**
*Random—complex conformality.*

### 3.4 Semiotic symptomatology: From observation to explanation/interpretation

Deriving from a non-therapeutic/non-pathological approach to autism, we will be focusing on our semiotic-symptomatic frame in two directions:

#### *3.4.1 The semiotic symptomatic dimension: Explanation and interpretation*

We, prior to any consideration, would like to make a relevant distinction between the symptomatic duality on the spectral space and its semiotic output on ($n$-1) meaning level in which the point at infinity [56] and bidirectionality (axiom of direction) are enabled. We call this level the meaning-translatum of the knowing field. Given complex/real parts of this plane, a projection principle will preserve the same considerations of the real part, except the spheric object (Riemannian sphere).

### 3.5 Prior to both

The symptomatic dimension of the object, its variability can only be semiotically defined if the object for which it studies meaning type is defined. Thus, without expression/content variability on the knowing/knowable object, there is no meaning possible and only description/definition, function … .

From semiotic/semiological directions, we define expression/content levels of the symptomatic principle. In addition, sequencing propositions for the latter (their coordinates), in particular the embedding of a linguistic into a non-linguistic individual is not a one-to-one equivalence (not injective). Moreover, we reconsider expression/content classical terms to belong to a non-directional frame of meaning. Dimension two functions of semiosis do not address the object for which they map meaning relations if:

- It does not specify polarity of its mapping (content-to-expression/expression-to-content).
- It lacks acts/facts of the scientific object.
- It lacks the directional meaning of the symptomatic point.

In this regard, a rewriting taking into consideration (*n*-1 level) translata algorithms of meaning is adopted. Henceforth, from D2 duality on explanation, we define *sequence connectivity* as meaning operators on embedded sequences within the field. To distinguish these sequences, we apply the following principle:

- Participational sequences: autistic-autistic/autistic-non-autistic
- Non-participational sequences: autist alone.

We apply two distinction functions: first, a discrete binomial function (Probability mass function) on independent experiences (sequences) with success P = 1, failure (Q = 1-P),

$$\mathrm{f(k,n,p)} = \mathrm{Pr^{-}(X = k)} = \binom{n}{k} p^{k}(1-p)^{n-k} \tag{20}$$

Secondly, a hypergeometric function for a dependent condition.

On a random variable X,

$$\mathrm{P_x(k)} = \mathrm{P_r(X = k)} = \frac{\binom{K}{k}\binom{N-K}{n-k}}{\binom{N}{n}} \tag{21}$$

Therefore, the correlation and convolution (also covariance) of both discrete binomial function, hypergeometric function will define a sequencing principle on the spectrum.

*DOI: http://dx.doi.org/10.5772/intechopen.1010189*

### 3.6 Explanatory semiosis

In the sense of observational scientific semiotics, sequence connectivity [57], its scale refers to undirected graph edge/node connectivity within a construction testing separation and disconnectedness (cuts and other operations). Thus, lacking modular (self-referential) acts of the knowing (epi-dimension), expression level, as a component, targets herein the sense of symptomatic observation on the spectrum. Inversely, explanability refers to the status of the difference between diagnosis and observation from our considerations. Particularly, from individuals' spectrum (CEA). In terms of notations and symbols,

$$\text{Expl} = \frac{\Delta diag}{\Delta obind} \tag{22}$$

Or the change in variation of both. Explanability of the results enables us to define the symptomatic 2D of **Figure 18**.

Secondly, rewriting the translata requires an observational model that distinguishes between "objectal" and "subjectal" semiosis in the sense of scientific, non-anthropomorphic, particulate directionality. Another advantage is that translata are not changed by non-zero factors in the sense that

$$(x; y) = (\lambda x; \lambda y) \tag{23}$$

implying that the explanatory model of semiosis will not redundantly replicate objective dimensions of the spectrum.

- *Explanatory translata*

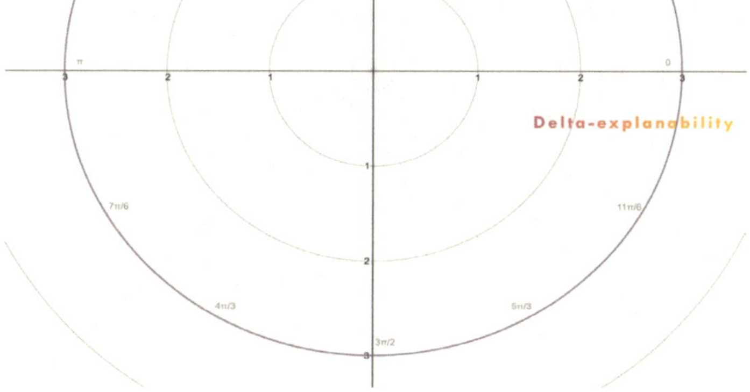


**Figure 18.**
*Explanation plane.*

Inferential applicability on the semiotic set of projection lines P over a field K, $P^1(k)$, therefore explanation additivity on two semiotic projective lines of homogeneous coordinates yields explanatory point calculus in the following sense:

$$[x_1 : x_2] + [y_1; y_2] = [(x_1y_2 + y_1x_2) : x_2y_2] \tag{24}$$

For which the semiotic explanation proposal would be:

$$[\text{low explanability} : \text{low edge connectivity}] \rightarrow$$
$$[\text{higher non} - \text{linguistic coherence} : \text{lower linguistic coherence}]$$

Yields a new point on spectrum condition

### 3.7 Interpretation semiosis

Plane inversion implies "subjectal semiosis" or direction change whereby node connectivity varies in respect of delta-interpretability. In this sense, delta-interpretability captures the ratio of the change in interpretation principles of both ROAL-approach and ASD diagnosis model adopted (or approach). Therefore, node connectivity will serve to refer to sequence adjacency within the graph, in terms of qualitative description or **Figure 19**.

Applying interpretive products from $P^1(k)$ on homogeneous points, we yield interpretive points

$$[y_1' : x_1'].[y_2' : x_2'] = [y_1'x_1' : y_2'x_2'] \tag{25}$$

For which the interpretation semiosis proposal will be written as an absorbing product of two interpretations with a different direction to explanation yielding a third interpretation point with polarity of loss or gain of interpretability.

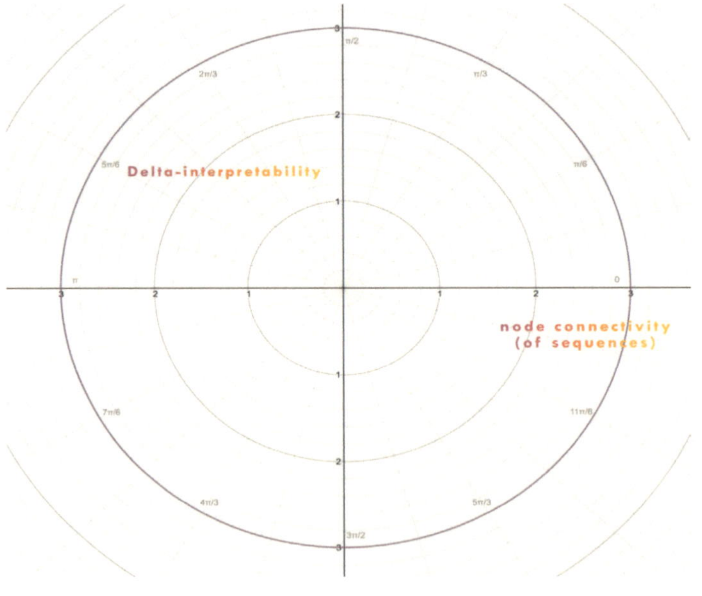


**Figure 19.**
*Interpretation plane.*

*DOI: http://dx.doi.org/10.5772/intechopen.1010189*

## 4. Conclusion

In this chapter, we have addressed a space conjecture and its knowing/knowable directions. In so doing, we started with an assumption of autism being viewed from an epistemic perspective, not through the lens of a pathological inquiry. This "stance" is not only due to our model of language nor is it due to the important distinction between symbolic and instrumental levels of language we owe Jakobson-Kurt, it derives from the need to avoid discrimination criteria used (or better said elimination methodology) by classical linguistics and structuralism. Instead of this tendency, we target the epistemic field in its nuances, especially from the double epi/meta perspective of double knowledge and the set of dual, representational notions belonging to the same condition. We have, therefore, an inversion of the neurotypical knowing field, thanks to a threefold methodological orientation.

- Investigating random; probabilistic dimensions, being a search for space and boundary order in the sense of an autistic inferential specificity of reasoning with the parameters of individuation.

- Investigating the epistemic, particulate shape of knowledge within mental/physical spaces through languages/individual language. Hence, an autistic spectral mode of search in which the notion of planar spectrum yields new directions on both parametrization and the status of individual language (individuation) in autism.

- The status of apperceptive individuality from individuation: in particular, hypo-hypersensitivity and its perceptual correlates (intero/proprio/extero) suggest the rereading of individuation invariants and exponents in the abovementioned sense. Therefore, we obtain a symptomatic "observable scene" where the interplay of perceptual spheres is the core object of language/autism data.

Secondly, the complexity of individuality/individuation and configuration within the field indicates the very point of the monistic thesis: in the horizon of interconnectivity, the autistic brain exhibits—through our conjecture—dimensional impairment (the cortical low dimensional manifold and its autistic challenge) properties where computational and number spaces are to be considered. Furthermore, the hypothetic "categorified" model of the autistic brain (hippocampal-cortical interactions) would rather suggest a transformation model whereby random spectral variance (this latter as an object) benefits from a particulate worldview where surfaces are patterned forms of probability measures (in particular, intervals) mapping this very search onto the spectral plane.

Autism proves to be an amnesic form of our knowledge, in that it shows an uncanny sense of variance and its abyssal non-configured space.

## Author details

Noury Bakrim
ILCS (Rabat), Morocco

*Address all correspondence to: bakrim_noureddine@yahoo.fr

## References

[1] Bakrim N. The biolinguistic instantiation: Form to meaning in brain/ syllable interactions. In: Silvera-Roig M, López-Varela A, editors. Cognitive and Intermedial Semiotics. London, UK: Intechopen; 2020. pp. 105-138

[2] Bakrim N. The Real-Object-Approach of Language (ROAL-Model): A Bio-Mathematical Attempt on Language and Consciousness. Paris: BoD; 2021a. 64p

[3] Bakrim N. Pour une linguistique de la double structuration réflexive (tome 1). Paris: BoD; 2021b. 88p

[4] Bakrim N. The Manifold Object of Language: A Bio-Mathematical and Socio-Mathematical Hypothesis from the ROAL-Model (3). Paris: BoD; 2022b. 68p

[5] Bakrim N. Spaces, Dimensions, Events: The Real Object Approach of Language - a Hypothesis on Language (along with a Text in French). Paris: BoD; 2024. 88p

[6] Boeckx C, Theofanopoulou C. A multidimensional interdisciplinary framework for linguistics: The lexicon as a case study. Journal of Cognitive Science. 2014;**15**:403-420

[7] Friedrich J. Psychopathology and the essence of language: The interpretation of aphasia by Kurt Goldstein and Roman Jakobson. History of Psychiatry. 2006; **17**(4):419-436

[8] Bakrim N. The Real-Object-Approach of Language (ROAL-Model): A Bio-Mathematical Attempt on Language and Consciousness. Paris: BoD; 2021a. p. 52

[9] Bakrim N. The Manifold Object of Language: A Bio-Mathematical and Socio-Mathematical Hypothesis from the ROAL-Model (3). Paris: BoD; 2022

[10] Buzsaki G. Rhythms of the Brain. Oxford: Oxford University Press; 2006. 465p

[11] Ingber D, Tensegrity I. Cell structure and hierarchical systems biology. Journal of Cell Science. 2003;**116**(Pt7):157-173

[12] Kanno Y. Topology optimization of Tensegrity structures under self-weight loads. Journal of Operations Research Society of Japan. 2012;**55**(2):125-145

[13] Beloussov L, Gordon R. Two ways for interpreting Driesch's law: "Positional information" and morphogenetic fields. Biosystems. 2018; **173**:7-9

[14] Spaulding EG. Driesch's theory of vitalism. The Philosophical Review. 1906;**15**(5):518-527

[15] Bühler K. (Trans. Goodwin D. F. & Eschbach, A.)Theory of Language: The Representational Function of Language. Amsterdam: John Benjamins Publishing; 2011. p. 570

[16] Noel J-P, Lytle M, Cascio C, Wallace TM. Disrupted integration of Exteroceptive and interoceptive signaling in autism Spectrum disorder. Autism Research. 2018;**11**(1):194-205

[17] Loureiro F, Ringold S, Lisa A. Interoception in autism: A narrative review of behavioral and neurobiological data. Psychology Research and Behavior Management. 2024;**17**:1841-1853

[18] Proff GL, Williams LQ, Garfinkel S. Sensory processing in autism across exteroceptive and interoceptive domains iris. Psychology & Neuroscience. 2022; **15**(2):105-130

[19] Chang H-L. Is language a primary modeling system? On Juri Lotman's

concept of semiosphere. Sign Systems Studies. 2003;**31**:2

[20] Keysers C, Gazzola V. Hebbian learning and predictive mirror neurons for actions, sensations and emotions. Philosophical Transactions of the Royal Society B. 2014;**369**:20130175

[21] Cuppini C et al. Hebbian learning mechanisms help explain the maturation of multisensory speech integration in children with autism Spectrum disorder (ASD) and with typical development (TD): A Neurocomputational analysis. Frontiers Human Neuroscience. 2012;**11**: 390-394

[22] Sotero R, Sanchez-Bornot J-M. Hebbian learning-guided random walks for enhanced community detection in correlation-based brain networks. In: Proceedings of Intelligent Data Engineering and Automated Learning (IDEAL é2023). Evora, Berlin: Springer; 2023. pp. 222-232

[23] Wikipedia. Available from: www.en.wikipedia.org/wiki/Natural_numbers_object [Accessed: November 1, 2024]

[24] Wikipedia. Available from: www.en.wikipedia.org/wiki/Riemann_zeta_function [Accessed: October 15, 2024]

[25] Bershadskii A. Hidden periodicity and chaos in the sequence of prime numbers. Advances in Mathematical Physics. 2011;**519178** 8 p

[26] Bakrim N. Spaces, Dimensions, Events: The Real Object Approach of Language - a Hypothesis on Language (along with a Text in French). Paris: BoD; 2024

[27] Fontanille F. Sémiotique du discours. Limoges: Pulim; 2003. 304p

[28] Duan X, Chen H. Mapping brain functional and structural abnormities in autism spectrum disorder: Moving toward precision treatment. Psychoradiology. 2022;**2**:78-85

[29] Rolls E-T, Deco G, Zhang Y, Feng J. Hierarchical organization of the human ventral visual streams revealed with magnetoencephalography. Cerebral Cortex. 2023;**33**:10686-10701

[30] Le Bihan D. On time and space in the brain: A relativistic pseudo-diffusion framework. Brain Multiphysics. 2020;**1**: 100016

[31] Chellig J, Fountoulakis N, Skerman F. The modularity of random graphs on the hyperbolic plane. arxiv: 2014.01041v1 [mathPR]; 2021

[32] Heggs et al. Neural manifold analysis of brain circuit dynamics in health and disease. Journal of Computational Neuroscience. 2023;**51**:1-21

[33] Kopell NJ. Beyond the connectome: The Dynome. Neuron. 2014;**83**(6): 1319-1328

[34] Brémaud N. Autisme: de bords à corps. L'Information psychiatrique. 2011;**87**:649-656

[35] Milnor J. Sommes de variétés différentiables et structures différentiables des sphères. Bulletin de la Société Mathématique de France. 1959; **87**:439-444

[36] Davermann R. Decompositions of Manifolds. Orlando: Academic Press; 1986. 331p

[37] Neklyudova A et al. Electrophysiological and behavioral evidence for hyper- and hyposensitivity in rare genetic syndromes associated with autism. Genes. 2022;**13**:671

[38] Zhang K. Imbalance of excitatory/inhibitory neuron differentiation in

neurodevelopmental disorders with an NR2F1 point mutation. Cell Reports. 2020;**31**(3):107521

[39] Arbib M. How the Brain Got Language: The Mirror System Hypothesis. Oxford: Oxford University Press; 2012. 432p

[40] Bakrim N. The biolinguistic instantiation: Form to meaning in brain/syllable interactions. In: Silvera-Roig M, López-Varela A, editors. Cognitive and Intermedial Semiotics. Rijeka, London, UK: Intechopen; 2020

[41] Ferrari PF, Tramacere A, Simpson EA, Iriki A. Mirror neurons through the lens of epigenetics. Trends in Cognitive Sciences. 2013;**17**(9):450-457

[42] May P. Symmetric monoidal categories and enriched categories. Available from: http://www.math.uchicago.edu/~may/MISC/Enriching.pdf [Accessed: October 25, 2022]

[43] Bourceux F, Stubbe I. Short introduction into enriched categories. In: Coecke B, Moore D, Wilce A, editors. Current Research in Operational Quantum Logic. Fundamental Theories of Physics. Vol. 11. Dordrecht: Springer; 2000

[44] Jungck J et al. Multiscale graph-theoretic modeling of biomolecular structures. In: Robeva R, Macauley M, editors. Algebraic and Combinatorial Computational Biology. Orlando: Acadamic Press; 2019

[45] Kreutz–Delgado K. arxiv: 0906.4835v1 [Math.OC]; 2009

[46] Wikipedia. Available from: www.en.wikipedia.org/wiki/Euler_angles [Accessed: October 10, 2024]

[47] Kreutz–Delgado K. arxiv: 0906.4835v1 [Math.OC]; 2009. p. 2

[48] Livan G, Novaes M, Vivo P. Introduction to random matrices: Theory and practice. arxiv: 1712.07903v1; 2017

[49] Bantang J, Lim M, Arielle Castro P, Monterola C, Saloma C. Foreign exchange market fluctuations as random walk in demarcated complex plane. arxiv: physics/0308062

[50] Klimenkova O, Menshutin A, Shchur L. Influence of the random walk finite step on the first-passage probability. arXiv:1712.02620v1 [cond-mat.stat-mech]; 2017

[51] Wikipedia. Available from: www:// en.wikipedia.org/wiki/Quantum_state [Accessed: December 15, 2024]

[52] Desbois J, Ouvry S. Numerical studies of planar closed random walks. arXiv:0804.1002v1 [cond-mat.stat-mech]; 2008

[53] Wikipedia. Available from: www.en.wikipedia.org/wiki/Brownian_Motion [Accessed: December 20, 2024]

[54] Lila G. Brownian motion in the complex plane (Kenyon summer science scholars program). Paper. 2014;**256**. Available from: http://digital.kenyon.edu/summerscienceprogram 256

[55] Markowsky G. Planar Brownian and complex analysis. arxiv, 2012. 08754v1 [Math.PR]; 2020

[56] Wikipedia. Available from: www.en.wikipedia.org/wiki/Projective_line [Accessed: December 25, 2024]

[57] Beineke L, Wilson R. Topics in Algebraic Graph Theory. Cambridge: Cambridge University Press; 2005. 293p